Your Midlife Body Code

Decode Symptoms, Realign the Body, and Reclaim Control

Claudine François

Aurora Corialis Publishing

Pittsburgh, PA

Printed in the United States of America

Edited by Allison Hrip, Aurora Corialis Publishing

Cover design by Karen Captline, BetterBe Creative

Paperback ISBN: 978-1-958481-62-2

Ebook ISBN: 978-1-958481-63-9

Praise for Your Midlife Body Code

"Claudine is the real deal. She truly understands what a woman's body needs to heal on a cellular level. Claudine is able to cut through the confusion and make sense of what's going on in a midlife woman's body. She really is master midlife body decoder!"
- Jenn Edden, Sugar Addiction Expert + Midlife Mental Health Coach

"I've spent countless hours trying to figure out why I didn't feel like myself, reading books, listening to experts, and digging through research. It was exhausting and often overwhelming. I only wish this book had existed back then. It would have saved me so much time and frustration. The content is spot on: clear, compassionate, and deeply insightful. It cuts through the noise and gets to the heart of what so many of us struggle with. If you've ever asked yourself, 'What's wrong with me?' this book might just be the answer you've been searching for."
- Melanie White, CEO, Hellwig Products, Inc.

"*Your Midlife Body Code* is a revelation! Every woman in their thirties, forties, and fifties **needs** this book. It is filled with practical, science-backed information and strategies that take the guesswork out of navigating perimenopause and menopause. The resources, worksheets, and information guides make it easy to put the Midlife Body Code into practice. I wish I had this amazing guide ten years ago, and I am grateful to have it now!"
- Jennifer Shepherd, AVP, Sales Manager, Chicago Title

"Midlife symptoms can feel confusing. One day it's fatigue, the next it's restless sleep or stubborn weight that won't budge. *The Midlife Body Code* makes sense of those patterns in a way that feels both validating and practical. What stood out to me is how clearly it explains that these struggles aren't just 'getting older,' but signals your body wants you to understand. Instead of offering quick fixes, it gives you tools and perspective that actually fit real life. Reading it felt like finally connecting the dots and realizing there's a better way forward."

- Krista Beavers, CEO & Founder, Guardian Accounting, Inc.

"*Your Midlife Body Code* is a game-changer for women who feel overloaded with advice from nutritionists, trainers, doctors, and social media trends, yet still struggle to make it work in real life. I wasn't chasing quick fixes; I had plenty of training that worked for me. What I lacked was a way to integrate it into a holistic lifestyle that truly lasts. This book gave me a clear, practical system that finally fits my body and my life. Claudine has created a roadmap for women to reclaim lasting health, energy, and balance in midlife and beyond."

- LeTasha Souffrant, Holistic Life Balance Coach

Table of Contents

Introduction: You're Not Crazy. You're Not Broken. You're Just Missing the Code.

A quick note before we start this party ...

Let's get real for a minute.

If you've picked up this book, chances are you're carrying a little extra weight that won't budge, no matter what you do. You're scattered, your brain feels foggy, like you're wading through molasses, forgetting words mid-sentence or zoning out mid-conversation. And, on top of it all, you're exhausted. Not just tired, but bone-deep drained, dragging yourself through the day, snapping at people you love, and lying awake at three a.m., wondering what the hell happened to your body (and your brain).

You've probably heard all kinds of explanations:

"It's just your age."

"It's stress."

"Your labs look normal."

But deep down, you know something's off. And you're right.

What you're feeling isn't made up, and it isn't just about hormones or aging. It's your body sending signals that it's stuck in survival mode. The problem is that traditional medicine isn't trained to decode those signals. But that's where this book and method come in.

Over the past several years, I've helped countless women uncover what's *actually* going on in their bodies using a clear, strategic process called **The Midlife Body Code** Method. It's a three-phase approach designed to help you move from confused and depleted to clear, energized, and thriving.

Each chapter in this book walks you through a specific aspect of that method. You'll get real answers, clear steps, and practical tools to help you reconnect with your body—and feel like yourself again.

Are you ready? Let's begin with what your body's been trying to tell you all along. I'll start with my own story, because this isn't just theory for me. I've felt the exhaustion, the frustration, and the *is this just aging?* doubts that creep in. That's why I know how deeply these struggles hit and why I believe they're not the end of the story.

From Corporate Powerhouse to Health Burnout

If you're like most women I know, you're making shizzle happen EVERY. DAMN. DAY. You've got the hustle. You're grinding it out. You're taking care of ALL the things from shuttling kids around to running a business, a department, or a household. Basically, you're superwoman.

And *being* superwoman is being the BEST. Right??

Because that's *exactly* what we're socialized to do: *all* the things for *all* the people, regardless of whether you "feel" like doing it and despite the toll it takes on your body.

I know this firsthand. As the chief financial officer in a multi-national corporation, I oversaw offices on both coasts and in a few countries. *I THRIVED on getting it DONE.* I was up at five a.m., on the treadmill or at a workout by five fifteen a.m., made the kids' lunches, got myself ready, and was at my desk by seven thirty a.m. It was *go* from the minute I sat down (as a California-based employee, I was already hours behind the East Coast and European offices). And let's not even talk about the toxic work environment—undermining, constant firefighting, and the classic *What does a blonde California girl really know about numbers?* undertone.

By the time I shut down for the day, I was wrung out. I'd barely make it home in time to kiss the kids goodnight before crashing into bed.

This was my life. ***And I hated it.***

I thought I wanted this. In my twenties, the hustle was exhilarating—the deadlines, the chaos, the adrenaline of crossing another thing off the list—it was all part of the ride. But when that rush becomes your default, your body eventually turns on the warning lights.

For me, the warning lights looked like chronic migraines, debilitating fatigue, and belly fat that wouldn't budge.

Migraines, Exhaustion, and the Belly Bulge

By my mid-to-late thirties, my body was kicking off warning lights left and right. Saturdays became migraine central. Do not touch me, do not look at me, and *for the love of* ... no lights! The migraines left me dry heaving, unable to function. Worst of all? My toddler wanted to climb into my arms, and I had absolutely nothing left to give. I was completely spent.

And then there was the fatigue and the belly fat. I looked like I had it all together (I hid it well). But inside, I was tanked. I leaned hard on caffeine and sugar. Thursday payment run? Starbucks. Afternoon deadline? Candy jar. Boss in town? Let's add cookies.

My team and I had the full buffet of energy "drugs" at the office. And they worked ... until they didn't. Blood sugar highs followed by crashing lows had me constantly chasing another hit. Foggy brain, sluggish thinking, dragging body—all on repeat.

I work out, I swear!

Despite my strict workout routine (strength training three times a week and cardio two to three times), the belly fat would not budge. I ate what I thought was healthy. I was doing everything "right," but it didn't matter. I was stuck in a cycle that wasn't working.

And when I went to my doctor, I hit a wall.

My job came with good health insurance, so I thought I'd take full advantage. At my annual check-up, I checked the box for migraines. She gave me meds. I threw them up. Next appointment: anti-nausea meds. Still didn't work. Her final solution? "Use the anti-nausea meds … from the bottom up." (Because apparently, when in doubt, there's always the suppository option?)

That's when I thought, *Why aren't we asking what's causing these problems?*

But to her, there was no cause. My labs were normal. Everything was "fine."

Except it wasn't.

The Promise of Western Medicine

Western medicine isn't trained to find root causes. It treats symptoms. You've got a problem? Here's a pill—or five. When one doesn't work, here comes another. It's whack-a-mole care.

For acute issues, Western medicine is top-notch. When I broke my foot, I went to Urgent Care. But for chronic issues, the traditional model falls short. That's not a dig; it's just not their training.

The Promise of Functional Medicine

Then I found someone in my town practicing a version of functional medicine. She ran three labs: a hair tissue mineral analysis (HTMA), a GI-map, and a food sensitivity panel. What we uncovered was blood sugar dysregulation, thyroid imbalance, and leaky gut.

Joy! Answers.

Most people wouldn't celebrate these results, but I did. Finally, someone wasn't telling me I was "fine." She said, "You've got stuff. But we can work with this." And just as importantly, she reassured me that it wasn't my fault. That I hadn't failed. I'd just been missing the right map.

We were **decoding** *my body's messages.* My symptoms weren't annoyances; they were information. Once I learned to read them, everything changed.

Why Midlife Women Are Struggling (and Being Ignored)

If you're reading this book, chances are you've also been gaslit: told it's normal, it's stress, or *just aging.* And to be fair, it's not always intentional. Most people (doctors included) have simply bought into the belief that this is what midlife *is supposed* to feel like. Maybe you've all but given up trying to get answers. Maybe you've blamed yourself. Maybe you've been told to just eat less and exercise more, *even* when you're eating 1,000 calories a day and crushing every high-intensity interval training (HIIT) workout.

It's exhausting. It's maddening. *And it is not OK.*

These are the routine responses:

- You're exhausted? *Sleep more or "manage your stress."*
- Can't lose weight? *Try fasting!*
- No libido? *Try lingerie or role play (seriously?!).*
- Still feel like shizzle, but your labs are normal? *Must be in your head ...*

Here's the truth: It is NOT normal to feel this drained, foggy, inflamed, and disconnected from your body. And it is *definitely* not just stress or aging. What you're experiencing is a mismatch between what your body needs and the kind of support you're getting. With the right tools, you can change that.

You Don't Always Have to Be the Strong One

You're the one everyone leans on—the glue that holds everything together. You're capable. You're the fixer. But that doesn't mean you don't get to take care of *you*.

Being the strong one doesn't mean you are invincible. That "cortisol rush" you've been running on for years? It's likely drained your body's resources and left you wired, tired, and running on empty.

And even though you look high-functioning on the outside—still showing up, still doing the things—you're unraveling inside. *You're holding it together with coffee, willpower, and a mountain of supplements.*

But here's the thing: It doesn't have to be this hard. And it shouldn't be.

Stuck in Survival Mode

Most women I work with don't even realize they're stuck in survival mode. It's just become their default:

- No energy at night for hobbies or connection because they're just trying to make it to bedtime
- Too tired to function but can't sleep because they're wired and restless
- Wide awake at three a.m. with a racing mind and an endless to-do list

When they finally seek help, they're handed a prescription or told their labs are fine.

This is what midlife women are experiencing. Not because they're broken but because the system is. Those outdated models of "care" aren't helping. And it's time we stopped pretending they are.

Why Traditional Advice Is Failing Us

If you've ever followed a diet or workout plan to a "T" but still felt exhausted, foggy, and puffy, it's not because you weren't *trying* hard enough. Midlife bodies are different. You can't just "power through" hormone shifts, nervous system dysregulation, mineral depletion, or gut dysfunction. Your metabolism didn't tank because you got lazy. It's reacting to a perfect storm of internal stressors and a lack of key resources.

The old advice, "eat less, move more," wasn't built for women navigating perimenopause, chronic stress, and burnout. What you need now isn't more willpower; it's a different strategy.

A strategy that helps you decode what's actually going on, realign your body with what it needs, and reclaim the energy, resilience, and joy that's still inside you.

Symptoms Are Signals, Not Annoyances

If you're dealing with frustrating symptoms, please know this: I'm not downplaying your pain. But your symptoms are *not* the enemy. They're the only way your body can speak to you.

Remember those debilitating migraines I used to get every weekend? They were my body's desperate attempt to get my attention. Your symptoms—whether it's joint pain, digestive issues, skin problems, brain fog, PMS, stubborn weight, or anything else—are doing the same. They're signals.

So, here's a mindset shift: What if the thing you've been trying to get rid of—the very thing you've been blaming yourself for—is actually the key to understanding what your body needs?

- Your body isn't broken; it's *brilliant*!
- It's not sabotaging you; it's sending you signals.
- It's not trying to make your life harder; it's *begging* for your attention.

And if you can learn to listen with the right tools, everything changes.

Knock, knock.

Who's there?

(You know the joke ...)

Knock, knock.

Who's there?

Hormone.

Hormone who?

Hormone reason to skip the gym today—I need a nap and a snack! ;)

Back to real talk: Those "knocks" are your body's notifications. It's saying, *Hey—something's off.*

Some examples:

- Exhaustion might be a sign of blood sugar issues, adrenal depletion, or gut imbalance.
- Bloating could mean low stomach acid or a stressed-out nervous system.
- Brain fog might signal that your minerals are low or inflammation is affecting your gut-brain axis.
- Irritability could point to hormone imbalances or a nervous system stuck in overdrive.

Symptoms aren't annoyances. They're clues. When you start treating them like messages—not moles to whack down—you take back your power.

That's the shift.

This is *your* Midlife Body Code—and it's learnable.

Every woman's body has its own language. And just like learning Spanish or French, you can learn yours. Once you understand the patterns and decode the messages, you stop guessing and *start* responding with what your body truly needs.

The **Midlife Body Code** is about helping you *decode those messages and realign your body* with what it *actually* needs so you can reclaim your energy, clarity, metabolism, and mood.

You'll stop asking, *What's wrong with me?*

And start asking, *What is my body asking for right now?*

The Promise of This Book: A Practical Codebreaker for Your Body

And that is *exactly* what you will learn in this book: how to decode your body's symptoms to get the health back that you *deserve*. This is not another *lose weight fast!* message or any other gimmick that leaves you burned out, bloated, and starving before landing you right back where you started. And it's definitely not a *Let's try thinking positively (and ignore what's going on in the body)* book either.

If you're like most of the women I know and have worked with, you've tried the detoxes, the calorie counting, eating two hundred grams of protein, *not* eating, just "pushing through" at whatever crazy workout is trending ... and if any of that had actually worked long-term, you wouldn't be here.

*This is a strategic, compassionate guide to **taking your power back**.*

This is about making the connection between what you are *feeling* in your body and what you can *do* about it. It is about understanding why it feels like your body is turning against you and learning how to work *with* it, rather than *against* it.

You'll get a step-by-step framework that explains what's going on under the surface, shows you how to identify and interpret your symptoms, and gives you *real tools* (that work for *your* life) to start feeling like yourself again.

You'll stop guessing and start decoding.

By the time you finish this book, you'll know how to:

- Read your body's signals instead of just bandaging them

- Connect the dots between fatigue, mood swings, digestive woes, weight fluctuations, and deeper imbalances
- Support your metabolism, hormones, nervous system, and gut—without the fad diets or workouts

This isn't about "doing it all." It's about doing *what works for your body, NOW*, driven by what your body *actually needs*, not outdated advice.

Not some perfect version of you.

Not your twenty-five-year-old self.

YOU—clear, energized, grounded, and strong.

I will show you how to decode, realign, and reclaim your body.

This isn't just a framework for this book; it's a process you can carry with you for life.

Phase 1: Decode

We'll uncover the hidden root causes behind your fatigue, brain fog, stubborn weight, cravings, and mood swings, even if your labs say you're "fine." You'll start learning how to read your body's signals and spot the patterns that matter most.

Phase 2: Realign

We'll restore the systems that have gone off course, like blood sugar balance, digestion, mineral status, and your nervous system. No extreme diets, punishing workouts, or overflowing supplement drawers required—just smart, strategic support.

Phase 3: Reclaim

This is where you rebuild trust with your body. You'll know what it needs, and it will respond. Your energy, mood, and metabolism start working with you, not against you, because you've given your body the tools it's been asking for all along.

That's **Your Midlife Body Code**. And by the end of this book, it's going to be *your personal* code. One you can come back to anytime life throws you out of whack.

Let's be honest: Midlife isn't the end; it's the moment you reclaim the narrative, step into your power, and create a story that actually honors who you are.

How to Use This Book

This isn't a "read it once and forget it" kind of book. It's designed to be a practical tool—one you can highlight, dog-ear, and come back to again and again. Each chapter gives you actionable insights and steps to try right away. Go in order or start where your symptoms are loudest. Either way, this is *your* toolkit, so use it in whatever way works best for YOU!

You'll also notice optional bonus tools and resources sprinkled throughout the book. These are for you to explore if you want to go deeper on a specific topic or need extra support in an area that's especially relevant to you. You don't need to stop and work through them before moving on. They're there whenever you're ready! I've also included them in a resource page at the end of the book, in case any section is *too long*, and you *didn't read* (TL;DR)!

I'm so glad you're here! Let's get started.

TL;DR—Introduction: You're Not Crazy. You're Not Broken. You're Just Missing the Code

- My story reflects what so many midlife women go through: hustling, pushing, and looking "fine" on the outside while migraines, exhaustion, and stubborn weight pile up on the inside.
- Traditional medicine often offers pills or a "your labs are normal" brush-off but rarely the real answers women need. Functional medicine helps uncover what's happening beneath the surface.

- Midlife women are often dismissed—told it's aging, stress, or lack of willpower—when in reality their bodies are stuck in survival mode.
- Symptoms aren't annoyances or failures; they're signals from your body pointing to deeper imbalances.
- The Midlife Body Code Method gives you the framework to Decode, Realign, and Reclaim your energy, clarity, and resilience without fad diets, punishing workouts, or more willpower.

Bottom line: You're not broken; you're just missing the code. This book will help you find it.

Part 1: Decode

You've been told you're "fine" but you don't feel fine. You're exhausted. Foggy. Puffy. Crashing by three p.m. and snapping at the people you love.

This is where that ends.

In this section, we're going to decode what your body's been trying to tell you. Your symptoms aren't random, and they're definitely not your fault. They're messages. And once you know how to read them, you'll never see your body the same way again.

Because clarity isn't just power, it's the first step to getting your energy, your mood, and your body back on your side.

Chapter 1: When "Fine" Isn't Fine

If you've ever been told you're fine when you knew you weren't, this chapter is for you.

You're sitting in your doctor's office. You've just listed your symptoms: exhaustion, weight gain, heart palpitations, bloating, mood swings, and sleepless nights. You're hoping for answers, but they look at your labs and say, "Everything's fine."

And you want to punch them. Metaphorically, of course.

Because you sure as all get-out do *not* feel fine. (Feel free to insert your own "F" word, here.)

If you've had this experience, you're not alone. Every year, countless women walk into their doctors' offices with a laundry list of symptoms and leave with little more than a pat on the back.[1] Or worse, a prescription that doesn't address the real issue. And for women of color, the dismissal is even more pronounced.[2]

In my own practice, I've seen it all: antidepressants prescribed for insomnia, heart palpitations dismissed as "just stress," and of course, the "just lose weight" cure-all.

Unfortunately, this isn't surprising. A 2018 study published in *The Journal of Law, Medicine & Ethics* reported that women with pain are more likely to be seen as "hysterical, emotional,

---

[1] Maya Dusenbery, "Even Women Doctors Find Their Symptoms Aren't Taken Seriously," *Web*MD, April 9, 2022, https://www.webmd.com/women/features/women-doctors-symptoms-dismissed.

[2] Institute of Medicine (US) Committee on Understanding and Eliminating Racial and Ethnic Disparities in Health Care. Unequal Treatment: Confronting Racial and Ethnic Disparities in Health Care. Smedley BD, Stith AY, Nelson AR, editors. Washington (DC): National Academies Press (US); 2003. PMID: 25032386.

complaining ... and fabricating the pain, as if it is all in her head."[3]

I could barely write that sentence without wanting to throw something.

You're Looking at Her

I've been there. During the years when I was laid out by migraines and couldn't even keep water down, I was told everything looked "normal." But when your body is falling apart, that word—*normal*—feels like a slap in the face.

The disconnect between how I felt and what the labs said only deepened the frustration. Was I being dramatic? Imagining it? Losing my mind?

It felt dismissive, confusing, and completely isolating, especially when I was doing all the "right" things. And that's how so many of my clients feel when they first come to me: dejected, exhausted, and silently wondering if this might be their last shot at finally feeling like themselves again.

You're Not Alone

Let's call this what it is: gaslighting. And while it may not always be intentional, it's still damaging. You've probably heard one (or all) of these:

- "It's just stress."
- "That's normal for your age."
- "You just need to eat less and move more."
- "Maybe you should get more sleep."

---

3 Anke Samulowitz, Ida Gremyr, Erik Eriksson, Gunnel Hensing, "'Brave Men' and 'Emotional Women': A Theory-Guided Literature Review on Gender Bias in Health Care and Gendered Norms towards Patients with Chronic Pain," *Pain Research and Management,* February 25, 2018, https://doi.org/10.1155/2018/6358624.

Sound familiar?

When you hear those lines enough, you start to doubt yourself. You wonder if you're overreacting, not trying hard enough, or somehow to blame for the way you feel.

You're not.

None of this is your fault.

You're not crazy, lazy, dramatic, or weak.

You're dealing with real symptoms, and your body is trying to tell you something.

The problem isn't you. It's the system that's trained to look for disease, not dysfunction. The model that hands out vague advice and cookie-cutter solutions instead of taking the time to ask *why*.

It's not your fault that no one has helped you decode what your body's been saying all along.

That's why I created The **Midlife Body Code,** a method that helps you **decode** what your body's really saying, **realign** it with what it actually needs, and **reclaim** your energy, metabolism, and peace of mind.

Let's take a deeper look:

- **Decode:** Understand what your symptoms are *really* telling you and uncover the hidden imbalances standard labs miss
- **Realign:** Give your body what it's actually asking for—without punishing workouts, extreme diets, or guessing games
- **Reclaim:** Build a sustainable rhythm that brings your energy, mood, and metabolism back online so you can feel like *you* again

Here's a bit of truth serum: You don't need another cleanse, a hormone-balancing smoothie, or yet another round of "just get more sleep." You need a method that actually works for your midlife body. That's what this book is here to give you, and we'll walk through it together, step by step.

Now let's look at why so many traditional approaches miss the mark and how you can start reading the signs your body's been giving you all along.

Why Conventional Labs Often Miss the Bigger Picture

Standard labs are designed to catch *disease*, not *dysfunction*. They're like smoke detectors: They go off when there's a full-blown fire but stay quiet when there's just smoke smoldering in the walls. Your body could be compensating like crazy, keeping things "technically normal" while you feel anything but.

Here's what I mean:

- It's like rewashing the whites over and over again because they keep coming out pink ... instead of realizing there's a red sock hiding in the load.
- It's like turning the hose up to full blast when barely a trickle comes out, when what you *really* need to do is unkink the line.
- It's like pouring your third cup of coffee to push through the afternoon fog without ever asking why your brain crashes at two in the afternoon. (Hint: it's not just "getting older." Your blood sugar, cortisol, and minerals might be trying to get your attention.)

These are the kinds of "solutions" we're handed when we rely only on surface-level numbers. But the real power comes from spotting *patterns*, not just isolated lab values.

Bonus Tool: Symptom Decoder Guide

If your symptoms have felt random or confusing, I've created a tool that will help you start connecting the dots. It will help you learn how to map your symptoms to the deeper systems involved (like digestion, detox, blood sugar, or mineral balance), so you can stop guessing and start investigating what your body's trying to tell you.

Grab the bonus tool here: ☞ https://YourMidlifeBody Code.com/bonuses

Symptoms as Early Warning Signs

If no one's ever told you this before, your symptoms are not random, and they are *not* a personal failing. They are your body's built-in warning system, like the lights on your car's dashboard, and that system is working *exactly* as it should.

Fatigue is often the first warning your body gives you when something's "off."

Weight gain is not a lack of willpower. It's often your body's way of protecting you when your stress response is stuck in the "on" position.

Mood swings are not you being "hormonal." They are *biochemical feedback,* revealing that the delicate (and complicated) internal workings affecting your mood need attention.

You might even feel like your body has betrayed you. Like it's turned on you overnight. That's how one of my clients described it, and maybe you've used those exact words, too.

But what if it's not betrayal at all?

What if it's communication?

Your body is not broken. It's brilliant. And it's trying to get your attention.

These signals aren't meant to give you a guilt trip; they're meant to *guide you*. Just like the warning lights on your car can save you a *lot* of headaches if you pay attention to them and take the right steps, your body's signals can do the same. Once you start seeing them as messages rather than problems to fix, or bandage over, the entire narrative shifts.

That's where The **Midlife Body Code** comes in. Think of it as a way to reframe how you interpret what your body's saying—a more accurate, compassionate lens that helps you get real answers.

No more guessing.

No more self-blame.

Just knowledge.

And knowledge makes you *powerful*.

Real-Life Case Study: When "Everything's Fine" Isn't

One of my clients (we'll call her Janice) had a very similar experience. After seeing multiple doctors and running nearly every test under the sun, she came to me frustrated, inflamed, and over it. A serious athlete for most of her life, she couldn't understand why she suddenly felt so exhausted, puffy, achy, and foggy all the time. But since her labs were "normal," she kept hearing the same dismissive line: *"You're fine."*

Not even close.

When we started working together, we took a different approach. We ran a simple mineral test, checked in on her gut health, and looked at how her stress and hormone patterns were actually playing out in her body, not just on paper.

What we found explained *everything*. Her minerals were depleted, her thyroid was dragging, and her digestion was sluggish. There was real dysfunction beneath the surface, even though her conventional labs never picked it up.

One of the first things we did was add a basic adrenal cocktail—just sea salt, potassium, and lemon in water. Nothing fancy. But that one small shift gave her noticeably more energy each day.

And no, that drink didn't "fix" everything. But it was the first time in months that something actually helped, and it gave us the momentum to keep going.

Her labs may have been "normal," but her body was waving red flags. She just needed someone to help her decode the data.

You've Got This.

You've been told you're *fine*.

You've been told it's *normal*.

You've been told to try harder, do less, sleep more, stress less, eat cleaner, move more, be grateful, stop complaining, and—above all—accept that this is just "midlife."

But here's the thing: You're not crazy. Your body isn't rebelling against you. And this is not the time to give up!

The truth is your body isn't failing you; it's fighting *for* you. Every symptom, every signal, every crash and flare and foggy afternoon is your body's way of saying: *Pay attention.*

And now ... you are!

You're starting to see the cracks in a system that was never designed to support a woman like you—a driven, brilliant, high-capacity woman who has spent decades pushing through, showing up, and being everything to everyone ... until her body said *no more*. This book is your turning point. This is where things start to change.

Now, you're not just surviving.

You're investigating.

You're reclaiming your health with clarity, strategy, and power.

You're decoding.

And no, this won't be about chasing quick fixes or obsessing over perfect habits. It's about learning how to respond to your body with the respect it's always deserved.

In the next chapter, we'll unpack the "perfect storm" that's been brewing under the surface so you can stop blaming yourself for things that were never your fault in the first place.

Let's go.

TL;DR – Chapter 1: When "Fine" Isn't Fine

- Too many women are told "you're fine" when their labs look normal—even while they're exhausted, foggy, or struggling with stubborn weight, poor sleep, or mood swings.
- This dismissal often shows up as gaslighting: "it's just stress," "that's normal for your age," or "just lose weight"—leaving women doubting themselves, especially women of color.
- The truth is, standard labs are built to detect disease, not dysfunction. They miss the early imbalances your body is already signaling.
- Symptoms aren't overreactions or weaknesses; they're your body's warning lights, pointing to deeper issues that need attention.
- Once you start decoding those signals instead of ignoring them, you stop blaming yourself and begin reclaiming your health.

Bottom line: You're not broken; you're being misread. And once you learn how to decode what your body is communicating, everything starts to change.

Chapter 2: The Perfect Storm—Hormones, Nervous System, Blood Sugar, and Gut

Why is this happening now?

If you're like most of the women who come to me, you've had things dialed in for years. You knew exactly what to eat (and when), which workouts gave you the best results, and how to keep your energy, weight, and focus in check.

And then ... it all stopped working.

You used to be able to push through. You could eat the pizza, stay up late, have a glass (or two) of wine, crush your workouts, survive on stress, and still feel fine.

Now? You wish! Just *one* night like that leaves you bloated, exhausted, puffy, cranky, and wide awake at three a.m.

And you're thinking: *What alien took over my body? What changed?*

What You're up Against

What you're experiencing isn't random. And, contrary to what you may be hearing (*ad nauseum*), it's not *just* aging. It's the result of a *perfect storm* inside your body. Like a ripple effect, what used to be small, manageable changes are now adding up and overflowing into symptoms you can't ignore.

Think Thanksgiving dinner and you're the chef: You've got five pots on the stove, a turkey in one oven, a pie in the other, and everything needs your attention *right now*. One burner gets too hot, or something starts smoking, and suddenly it feels like it's all on the verge of chaos. That's midlife: every system demanding something at once, and you're trying to manage it all without burning out.

- **Your hormones are shifting** beyond the predictable twenty-eight-day cycle, throwing off sleep, mood, and metabolism.
- **Your nervous system is stuck in "survival mode,"** keeping you wired and tired while pushing everything else—hormones, digestion, detox, immune health—onto the back burner.
- **Your blood sugar is swinging wildly**, leading to stubborn weight (especially around the belly), energy crashes, cravings, and restless sleep.
- **Your digestion is slowing down**, so you're not breaking down food or absorbing nutrients the way you used to.
- **Your liver is overloaded** not just from wine or toxins but from excess hormones, gut overflow (like histamines), and stress byproducts it's trying to filter out.

Each of these might sound like a separate issue, but they're all connected. When one part tips out of alignment, it sets off a chain reaction that throws everything else off. It creates a snowball effect that leaves you feeling worse, even when you're "doing everything right."

You don't have to fix everything at once. You just need to see how these systems interact so you can stop guessing and start uncovering what's *really* behind your symptoms. You need to decode the pattern.

Let's break it down.

The Perfect Storm: What No One Told You About Feeling "Off"

1. Hormones: You're Gonna Miss Me When I'm Gone

Let's talk about hormones. We've all had a love/hate relationship with them, but midlife takes it to a whole new level. What used to be mildly annoying suddenly becomes full-on chaos.

I'm not here to give you a science lecture (though Alisa Vitti goes deep in on this topic in her book, *In the Flo,* if you're into graphs and hormone charts).[4] But what caused bloating, cramps, irritability, or heavy flows during your reproductive years is the same hormonal dance that can send you *off the rails* in midlife. It's like chaos on steroids.

Maybe the first sign is a wonky cycle. What used to be a predictable twenty-one to thirty-five days turns into a game of *When's it coming and how long will it last?* Then there's the bloating, fatigue, the random snappiness at people you love ... and the symptoms just keep stacking up. Like the proverbial frog in the pot of boiling water, you don't always realize how much has changed until everything feels wrong.

So, what's *actually* happening?

Let's define the basics:

- **Perimenopause** is the five to ten plus years leading up to menopause. (This is when the real rollercoaster begins.) It often starts in your late thirties or forties, but the timeline varies.
- **Menopause** is *one day* exactly twelve months after your last period.
- **Post-menopause** is everything *after* that.

---

4 Alisa Vitta, *In the FLO: Unlock Your Hormonal Advantage and Revolutionize Your Life* (HarperOne, 2020).

Women of color often experience symptoms *earlier* and for *longer* than their white counterparts.[5] And if you've had a hysterectomy, chemo, or certain procedures like ablation or IUD placement, your shifts may be more abrupt or harder to track.

Experts like Dr. Mary Claire Haver and Tamsen Fadal have outlined how perimenopause can impact everything from mood and metabolism to digestion, sleep, libido, and even skin, hair, and joints. If it feels like "everything" is shifting. You're not imagining it.[6]

Want a deeper look at your symptoms?

Download the **Midlife Load Tracker** at https://YourMidlifeBodyCode.com/bonuses or via the QR code below.

And here's the kicker: Many women go to their doctors for help and are dismissed or misdiagnosed.

---

[5] Siobán D. Harlow, Sherri-Ann M. Burnett-Bowie, Gail A. Greendale, *et al.*, "Disparities in Reproductive Aging and Midlife Health between Black and White women: The Study of Women's Health Across the Nation (SWAN)," *Women's Midlife Health* 8, 3 (2022), https://doi.org/10.1186/s40695-022-00073-y.
[6] Mary Claire Haver, *The New Menopause: Navigating Your Path Through Hormonal Change with Purpose, Power, and Facts* (Rodale Books, 2024); Tamsen Fadal, *How to Menopause: Take Charge of Your Health, Reclaim Your Life, and Feel Even Better Than Before* (Grand Central Publishing, 2025).

So, what's really going on?

Estrogen and progesterone start fluctuating in perimenopause, then drop for good at menopause. Here's how those shifts show up:

- **Sleep:** As progesterone drops, deep sleep gets harder. Cue the three a.m. wake-ups and restless nights. And when sleep goes, so does everything else: mood, cravings, focus, energy.
- **Mood stability:** Estrogen boosts serotonin (happiness) and dopamine (pleasure and motivation). Progesterone helps make GABA, that calming, "I've got this" chemical. When these decline, you're more anxious, snappy, wired, and overwhelmed. You're not "too emotional," you've just lost your hormonal buffer.
- **Hot flashes + puffiness:** Estrogen helps your brain regulate temperature. When it drops, your internal thermostat starts glitching—hello hot flashes, night sweats, and that "skin crawling" sensation. Progesterone usually backs it up, but when *both* are down, that heat dial gets stuck on high.
  Estrogen and progesterone usually keep inflammation in check. Without them, inflammatory messengers (like cytokines) can go wild, triggering more joint pain, bloating, and flare-ups than you're used to.
- **Metabolism:** Hormonal shifts mean less muscle and more fat storage, especially around the belly. Estrogen controls *where* fat goes. Progesterone supports your thyroid. When both drop, your body becomes a weight-storage machine that resists your usual efforts.

And then there's **testosterone**. This hormone isn't just about libido—it helps drive energy, focus, and muscle tone. It doesn't always tank in midlife, but chronic stress can drag it down. Support your nervous system, and you help testosterone hold strong. Protect your testosterone and you protect your energy, your edge, and that "get-stuff-done" mojo.

Why does this matter?

These aren't "just hormones." They influence every system in your body. Understanding their ripple effects is the first step to getting ahead of your symptoms instead of constantly chasing them down.

2. Nervous System Overdrive: The Silent Driver of Symptoms

You're trying to hold it all together: work, family, deadlines, hormones, aging parents, and the nightly question of what's for dinner. On the outside, it might look like you're doing a decent job, but on the inside, your body is bracing for impact.

That's your nervous system talking.

Most of us think of stress as something we *feel*—overwhelm, anxiety, irritability. But often the real stress response is happening underneath the surface. Your nervous system is like your body's operating system, always scanning for safety or threat. When it's stuck in fight-or-flight mode (aka sympathetic dominance), everything else gets pushed to the back burner.

Your digestion slows down. Your hormones get sidelined. Your metabolism flatlines. Even your immune system goes quiet. Because when your body thinks you're under threat, its job is to survive—not to thrive. This is why so many women in midlife feel like they're falling apart, even when they're doing "everything right."

Let's be clear: Your nervous system isn't busted. It's just exhausted from living in high alert. You've probably been pushing through for years, running on cortisol and caffeine, surviving on six hours of sleep, multitasking like a pro, and calling it normal. But now, your body is waving the white flag.

Here's the kicker: You can't out-supplement a frazzled nervous system.

No amount of magnesium, adaptogens, or ashwagandha will override a body that doesn't feel safe. Healing can't happen in fight-or-flight. The good stuff—digestion, hormone production, fat burning, deep sleep—it all happens when your body feels calm, grounded, and safe. That's called parasympathetic mode (or rest-and-restore).

This doesn't mean you need to meditate for ninety minutes or book a silent retreat. It means weaving *micro moments of safety* into your day. Try these:

- Take three deep belly breaths before meals
- Take two minutes of quiet while you sip your coffee
- Step outside and let the sun hit your face
- Turn off notifications for fifteen minutes and do *nothing*
- Say "no" to something that drains you (yes, it counts)

These little moments might not look like much, but to your nervous system, they're everything. They tell your body, *You're safe now. We can shift gears.*

And when that shift happens, everything else works better.

Still not sure what's draining you?

Download the **Midlife Load Tracker** at https://YourMidlifeBodyCode.com/bonuses to get a clearer picture. It will help you see what you've been carrying (even the invisible stuff), so you can finally start to lighten the load.

The connection is simple: When you weave small moments of safety into your day, your nervous system shifts out of survival mode. And that's when your energy starts to return. Cortisol (your main stress hormone) raises your blood sugar. That means every time your nervous system is in overdrive, your blood sugar is too, whether you've eaten a donut or not. You could be eating the cleanest meals of your life, but if your body is stuck in survival mode, it's going to spike your blood sugar anyway.

That's the loop so many women get stuck in, and why the next section matters so much.

Let's talk about how to balance your blood sugar (and your energy) without going low-carb, cutting out all the fun, or making things harder than they already are.

3. Blood Sugar Blues: The Problem You Didn't Know Existed

You're eating healthy, skipping snacks, maybe even intermittent fasting—and yet, you still feel exhausted, foggy, and stuck with the same stubborn weight. Here's what's really going on "under the hood."

The Hormone Connection

You might be wondering why we are spending so much time on hormones. Here's why: They affect everything, including your blood sugar.

- **Estrogen supports insulin sensitivity**. When estrogen dips in perimenopause, your body becomes less efficient at moving glucose out of the bloodstream and into your cells for energy. Translation: Even the "clean" foods you're eating might be stored as fat—particularly around the belly—because your cells aren't responding to insulin as effectively as before.
- **Progesterone helps buffer the stress response**. As progesterone drops, cortisol, the stress hormone, can spike more easily. And guess what cortisol does? It signals the liver to release glucose into your bloodstream, elevating blood sugar ... *even if you haven't eaten.* That sets you up for a crash later, especially if you're under-fueled.

The Rollercoaster Effect

Here's the real issue: the swing.

As Dr. Casey Means explains in her book, *Good Energy,* blood sugar isn't just about sugar; it's about stability.[7] When your glucose levels spike and crash all day, it doesn't just tank your energy; it fuels inflammation. And inflammation is the root of nearly every chronic condition out there.

More immediately, though, these glucose spikes lead to **insulin surges**. Over time, repeated surges wear out your cells'

---

[7] Casey Means (with Calley Means), *Good Energy: The Surprising Connection Between Metabolism and Limitless Health* (Avery / Penguin Random House, 2024).

sensitivity, leading to **insulin resistance**—a huge reason why it's harder to lose weight in midlife, even when you're eating well.[8]

What's Making It Worse?

You're not eating cake and cookies all day (I see you). Ironically, it's what you're *not* eating that's often the problem. For instance:

- Skipping meals or undereating protein and fat
- Cutting carbs too low, especially when your stress is high
- Going too long without food

Ironically, these are the very strategies diet culture promotes, and they're working against you.

The result?

- Afternoon crashes (you're not lazy, you're under-fueled)
- Brain fog, anxiety, or irritability when hungry (aka hangry)
- Wake ups from two to four a.m. when your blood sugar dips and your body pumps out cortisol to compensate
- Stubborn weight, bloat, and exhaustion, even with "clean" meals

Why This Matters

Here's what most women don't realize: Every blood sugar crash is a stress event. And every time your body crashes, it sends up the Bat Signal for cortisol. But when cortisol is "on," everything else gets pushed to the background: digestion slows,

---

[8] Natalia Matulewicz, Monika Karczewska-Kupczewska, "Insulin resistance and chronic inflammation," *Postepy Hig Med Dosw* (Online) 70(0) (2016): 1245-1258, https://pubmed.ncbi.nlm.nih.gov/28026827/.

hormones get sidelined, thyroid function dips, immune defenses go offline. When blood sugar swings become frequent, it's one of the first ways your systems begin to unravel, even if you're a healthy eater.

Over time, this constant internal SOS leads to what we call adrenal burnout. That's when your stress response becomes unreliable, leaving you drained, foggy, and disconnected from your own motivation.

Blood sugar is foundational.

When it's steady, everything else—mood, sleep, cravings, energy, hormones—stabilizes too. When it's not? It's like trying to build your health on quicksand.

And no, this isn't about avoiding carbs or tightening your diet. It's about **fueling your body consistently**, so it stops sounding the internal alarm all day (and night) long.

4. Gut Check: When Good Food Isn't Enough

Bloating. Brain fog. Random food sensitivities. You cut the gluten, ditched the dairy—so why does your gut still feel like a hot mess? ¿!Que pasa?! (What's happening?)

As someone who spent *years* cleaning up her gut, I can tell you this is a *big* part of your overall health. We've been spending a lot of time on hormones, and for good reason, but all the interventions in the world can't get you back on track if your gut is in a state of disrepair. And vice versa! These two functions are very tightly intertwined.

The Hormone-Gut-Stress Triangle

Believe it or not, estrogen and progesterone play a much bigger role in the gut than is often discussed. Estrogen supports gut motility (i.e., how well things move along the digestive tract), and progesterone helps keep inflammation down and supports tight junctions in the gut lining (when the junctions are *not* tight, that can be the beginning of "leaky gut").[9] So, when they both drop, you're in for a doozy! You may notice more bloating, sluggish digestion, and random sensitivities, even to foods you used to tolerate just fine!

And guess who's back to make this whole situation worse? That's right, chronic stress! Add to this mix some extra stress (Remember, with lower hormones, we're more sensitive to stress.), and not only is our mood impacted, but it's throwing off our digestion at every level:

- **Stomach acid drops**, making it harder to break down food. The result: indigestion, nutrient deficiencies, and if it happens often enough, a direct path to leaky gut.
- **Bile production slows**, making it harder to process and digest fats (which we need for hormones and brain function) and some key vitamins like A, D, E, and K. Plus, bile helps eliminate toxins and excess hormones. So, if it's not around to do the job, those waste products may be recirculated.
- **Pancreatic enzymes** take a vacation, too, so proteins and carbs don't get broken down or absorbed as well, either. And we need those things to fuel our bodies!

When cortisol is on, digestion is off. Your body isn't prioritizing bile, enzymes, or stomach acid when it thinks you're in danger. It's trying to survive, not break down lunch.

Here's the other rub: Lower progesterone means lower microbial diversity (the "good" bacteria), and that lack of good guys on our team means it's easier for the "bad guys" to come to the party. Coupled with cortisol turning "off" stomach acid and

---

9 Brandilyn A. Peters, Nanette Santoror, Robert C. Kaplan, Qibin Qi, "Spotlight on the Gut Microbiome in Menopause: Current Insights," *International Journal of Women's Health,* (2022):1059-1072, https://pubmed.ncbi.nlm.nih.gov/35983178/.

immune function, it creates the ideal environment for opportunistic bacteria, yeast, parasites, and other gut bugs.

And guess what happens when the party in our gut goes sour? It can trigger cravings, fatigue, and inflammation *and* negatively impact your mood (because eighty to ninety percent of the "feel good" neurotransmitters are made in the gut), and your hormones. In short: *no bueno* (not good).

Figure: The Midlife Chaos Loop

The hormone–gut–stress triad isn't just a list of symptoms; it's a feedback loop. Each system influences the others, creating a self-perpetuating cycle that leaves you feeling wired, inflamed, and exhausted. The upside is that once you spot the pattern, you can start breaking it.

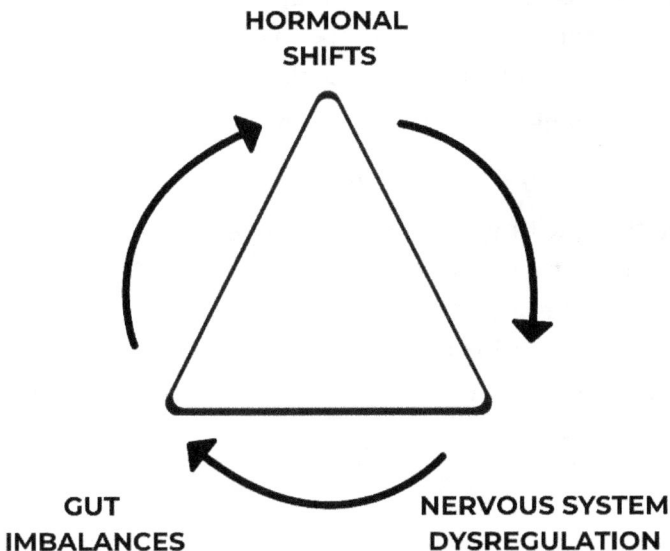

HORMONAL
SHIFTS

GUT
IMBALANCES

NERVOUS SYSTEM
DYSREGULATION

How And Where Symptoms Emerge
When Balance Breaks Down

Don't be like Britney—Overexposed and Toxic.

Toxins are *everywhere*: in our food, water, air, and yes, even our brains. One study recently found **microplastics lodged in human brain tissue**.[10]

No, you can't escape every toxin. But you *can* reduce your load and protect your gut in the process.

Here's where most women unknowingly sabotage themselves:

- Long-term use of antibiotics
- NSAIDs like ibuprofen or aspirin
- Hormonal birth control
- Ultra-processed "healthy" snacks or bars

These weaken the gut lining, kill off good bacteria, and pave the way for the "bad guys" (think yeast, pathogens, parasites) to take over. Over time, that creates the perfect storm for leaky gut, inflammation, and a whole-body cascade of symptoms.

The List of Symptoms Might Surprise You

The thing with symptoms of gut dysfunction is that you may not think of them as gut-related. I know I certainly didn't connect my migraines with my leaky gut from eating gluten or dairy with my cystic acne! Because it's not just gas or poop problems. Gut dysfunction shows up in every system of the body:

---

[10] Alexander J. Nihart, Marcus A. Garcia, Eliane El Hayek, et al., "Bioaccumulation of microplastics in decedent human brains," *Nature Medicine* 31, (2025): 1114–1119, https://doi.org/10.1038/s41591-024-03453-1.

- Bloating after meals
- Constipation *or* diarrhea
- Sudden food sensitivities or histamine reactions
- Skin issues (rashes, acne, eczema)
- Joint pain or stiffness
- Brain fog, fatigue, or irritability
- Pain between shoulder blades
- Insomnia
- Nausea

Do any of those stand out to you?

Why This Matters

The truth is, you can eat all the kale and quinoa in the world, but if your gut isn't breaking it down and absorbing it, your body is running on fumes. What's worse is that every meal could be triggering more inflammation if your gut lining is damaged or leaky.

Bottom line: If your gut isn't working, nothing else will. Not your hormones. Not your energy. Not your brain. Fixing your gut isn't just a "health" move; it's the foundation for everything that comes next.

Wrapping It Up—None of This Is Random

At this point, you've seen how midlife throws more than just a curveball—it throws you several. Hormones shift. Blood sugar gets unstable. Your nervous system runs in overdrive. And then digestion slows and food that used to be fine suddenly makes you feel like a balloon. None of these symptoms are happening in isolation. They're part of a larger conversation your body has been trying to have with you.

And when you use the **Midlife Load Tracker** to step back and look at the big picture, patterns start to emerge. What once felt random or unrelated suddenly clicks: *Ohhh ... no wonder I'm exhausted by three p.m. No wonder I'm bloated no matter what I eat. No wonder I feel like I could cry or bite someone's head off and have no idea why.*

This isn't about chasing symptoms. It's about decoding them.

Real Life: Hannah's Story

Hannah was in her mid-fifties when she came to me feeling like a stranger in her own body. She was tired all the time. Her digestion was off. She had a history of fatty liver and high cholesterol. And, although she ate well, she couldn't lose a pound. Her sleep was wrecked, especially around three a.m., and anxiety kept her mind racing at night. On paper, she looked "fine." In reality, her systems were struggling to keep up with the demands of midlife.

We didn't overhaul everything at once. Instead, we zoomed out. We simplified her meals to stabilize blood sugar, supported her liver to offload toxins and excess hormones, brought in mineral support for energy, and introduced daily "micro-reset" moments to help shift her nervous system out of survival mode.

Within a few weeks, she was sleeping through the night again. Her digestion smoothed out, the puffiness in her face and hands started to fade, and her anxiety began to quiet. Over time, her body stopped bracing and started releasing. She lost eighteen pounds, not because she chased weight loss, but because her body finally felt safe enough to let go.

Most importantly, she got her spark back. That's what happens when you stop pushing and start listening.

You're Not Broken

You're not crazy. You're not lazy. And you're definitely not broken. You're just dealing with a body that's been trying to adapt to a whole lot of change with very little support.

This chapter gave you the aerial view. Now, it's time to zoom in. In the next chapter, we'll take a closer look at one of the most overworked, misunderstood players in your midlife story: your liver.

And trust me, it deserves the spotlight.

TL;DR – Chapter 2: The Perfect Storm— Hormones, Nervous System, Blood Sugar, and Gut

- What you're experiencing in midlife isn't "just aging." It's a perfect storm of shifting systems all colliding at once.
- Hormone changes—especially dips in estrogen, progesterone, and sometimes testosterone—disrupt sleep, mood, metabolism, and inflammation.
- A nervous system stuck in survival mode keeps your body wired, drains your energy, and sidelines digestion, detox, and hormone balance.
- Blood sugar swings, often from under-fueling or stress, trigger fatigue, cravings, three a.m. wake-ups, and stubborn weight—even with healthy meals.
- Gut function slows as stomach acid, bile, and enzymes decline, paving the way for nutrient gaps, food sensitivities, leaky gut, and whole-body inflammation.

Bottom line: Midlife isn't about one thing going wrong; it's about multiple systems going off-track at the same time. The good news is that these patterns can be decoded. And, once you see them, you can finally do something about it.

Chapter 3: Your Liver's Cry for Help—The Hidden Load You're Carrying

If your liver can't keep up, neither can you.

So far, we've explored what's shifting in your hormones, blood sugar, and nervous system, but there's one major player we haven't given its full spotlight yet: your liver.

I know what you're thinking: *My liver? Really? Isn't that just about drinking?*

Not even close.

If you've been doing everything right—eating clean, moving your body, taking the supplements—and still feel bloated, inflamed, sluggish, or stuck, your liver might be the reason why. It's your internal cleanup crew, hormone processor, blood sugar helper, and inflammation filter. And when it gets overloaded, everything else backs up too.

This chapter is about looking under the hood to understand what else might be quietly driving your symptoms ... and why no plan will work if your liver is underwater.

Learn to Love Your Liver (The Overwhelmed Hero)

In case you've never once thought of your liver (I certainly hadn't!), it's a freaking rock star. Imagine being able to simultaneously make dinner, be the family chauffeur, bust out all your work assignments, *and* scale Mount Everest. That's what your liver does Every. Damn. Day. Before lunch! Truly, I think it's the most productive and underappreciated organ in our body.

The problem is that we're asking it to do all those things while using crutches, seriously impairing its ability to get it all done. Let's talk about why and what we can do about it.

Why Midlife Overwhelms the Liver

Since we're talking about my favorite organ here, please don't mind if I gush. It is this huge-ass filter in our body, and we are giving it a *lot* to do: processing hormones, managing blood sugar, supporting digestion, and keeping our entire system balanced. On a *good* day, these functions can all happen. When you add up our current environment *plus* the extra pressures/burdens/stressors in midlife, the demands stack up, and the filter gets clogged. In order of increased burden (lowest to highest), below are the things that are tripping it up.

The Hidden Burdens of Meds, Birth Control, & Food Intolerances

You're doing your best: clean meals, consistent habits, maybe even a few supportive routines in place. But if your liver is overwhelmed, you might still feel puffy, foggy, or inflamed.

Here's why:

Long-Term Med Use Adds Up

Your liver has to process every medication you take. And while medications can absolutely be helpful—even necessary— they do increase the detox burden over time.

Common culprits include:

- **Painkillers (NSAIDs)** like ibuprofen, aspirin, or naproxen
- **Reflux meds** like antacids or proton-pump inhibitors
- **Antidepressants or anxiety medications** like SSRI's, benzodiazepines, SNRI's

- **Hormonal birth control**, including pills, patches, and IUDs

These can interfere with bile flow, deplete key nutrients needed for detox and, especially in the case of hormonal birth control, add synthetic estrogens your liver has to work overtime to clear.

Food Intolerances & Gut Stress

Even when you're eating "clean," food intolerances can sneak in and stir up inflammation. And in midlife, this becomes more common, thanks to shifting hormones and a more sensitive gut lining.

You might suddenly react to foods that never bothered you before, like:

- Gluten or dairy
- Soy, corn, or eggs
- Histamine-rich or additive-laden packaged foods

When your body flags a food as a threat—even if it's something totally normal like eggs or spinach—it kicks into defense mode. Your immune system grabs the "invader," wraps it in a little histamine bubble (like a jail cell), and ships it off to the liver to deal with.

And the more that happens, the more cleanup your liver has to do. So, instead of focusing on hormone balance or clearing out toxins, it's stuck handling food fights all day. It's like trying to mop the floor while the sink is still overflowing.

And *this* is how gut issues become liver issues.

What This Means for You

Each of these factors—long-ago birth control, your daily meds, or that morning latte with a splash of dairy—might seem small on its own. But they're not happening in isolation. They're happening *on top of* everything else your liver is juggling: hormone detox, environmental toxins, blood sugar swings, and more. And when that system gets overloaded, symptoms start to show up ... even if you're doing "everything right."

And when estrogen doesn't clear the way it should, or inflammation stays high, you feel it in your energy, your mood, your skin, your sleep, and even your waistline.

The Buzz That Backfires: Alcohol & Caffeine

I hate to be the bearer of bad news, but if you're still trying to make wine and coffee work in midlife, your liver might be waving a white flag.

Alcohol: Not Worth the Trade-Off

Here's the truth: alcohol is *not* your friend right now. Even a little bit is a big ask for your midlife body.

Your liver has to drop everything to process it, which means hormone detox, nutrient conversion, and fat metabolism all get pushed to the back burner. And the worst part? Alcohol slows down estrogen clearance, making you more vulnerable to estrogen dominance, even if your estrogen is technically low. This shows up as things like mood swings, water retention, breast tenderness, belly fat, and irritability ... all from a glass or two.

Add in alcohol's effect on sleep (you might fall asleep fast, but you'll wake up around two or three a.m.) and the inflammation it fuels throughout the body, and it's just not worth it. Especially when your body is already working overtime.

Caffeine: Proceed with Caution

Caffeine gets a little more wiggle room but there's still a threshold. My rule of thumb? No more than **one cup a day** and preferably before noon.

Too much caffeine overstimulates the nervous system, jacking up cortisol and leaving your adrenals even more depleted. It's also a diuretic, which means you're flushing out the minerals your liver *needs* to function (like magnesium and potassium). That mid-afternoon coffee habit might feel like fuel, but it's quietly draining the reserves you're already low in.

And if you're feeling extra anxious, wired-but-tired, or struggling with sleep? That extra shot might be a bigger part of the problem than you think.

The Ripple Effect on Your Liver

In midlife, your body has a lower tolerance for hidden stressors. Alcohol and caffeine are two of the biggest ones, and while they may seem harmless, they're not happening in a vacuum. They're piling onto an already full plate, making it harder for your liver to do its job.

Cutting back (or cutting them out) isn't about deprivation; it's about making space for better energy, fewer symptoms, and the hormonal balance you've been working so hard to get back.

The Invisible Load: Environmental Toxins

You don't have to live near a chemical plant to be dealing with toxic exposure. It's in your makeup, lotion, detergent, candles, air fresheners, plastic containers, and even your receipts. And while your body is designed to handle *some* toxins, the problem today is the *sheer volume*, especially when your liver is already dealing with hormones, food reactions, meds, and blood sugar swings.

Midlife makes things trickier. Your detox pathways slow down, partly because your body isn't breaking things down or flushing them out as efficiently anymore. Suddenly, that lavender dryer sheet or plastic water bottle affects you differently, showing up as rashes, headaches, brain fog, fatigue, or even irritability or trouble sleeping.

And just because the symptoms are subtle doesn't mean they're harmless. These toxic compounds are known to:

- Disrupt hormones (especially estrogen)
- Fuel inflammation
- Burden the liver with more cleanup than it can reasonably handle

You can't control *everything*, but you can reduce your body's exposure by being choosy about what you put **on**, **in**, and **around** your body. Start with the things you use daily, like:

- Skincare and makeup (go fragrance-free when possible)
- Cleaning products (ditch the synthetic sprays and suds)
- Plastic water bottles and food containers (especially when heated)
- Scented candles, air fresheners, and dryer sheets (swap for essential oils and wool dryer balls)

Detox Your Products (Without Overhauling Everything)

Don't panic—this isn't about tossing out everything under your sink. But if you want to start making smarter choices for your body (and your liver), check out the Environmental Working Group's website, EWG.org, or their app. It's like a cheat sheet for cleaner living. Just search for your favorite products to see how they rank and start swapping the worst offenders first.

Why This Matters

Environmental toxins are a sneaky load. They don't feel heavy in the moment, but they add up fast. And when your liver gets bogged down from processing pesticides, plastics, and perfumes *on top of* hormones and food reactions, you feel it. In your skin, your energy, your mood, your weight.

Reducing that burden doesn't require perfection. You don't need to live in a bubble, just give your liver a little less mess to mop up. Your body will thank you.

The Hormone Detox Dilemma

Your liver plays a major role in processing hormones, especially estrogen. In midlife, as estrogen and progesterone levels fluctuate, your body produces more hormone metabolites that need to be cleared efficiently. But if your liver is already working overtime (thanks to years of stress, medications, processed foods, or chemical exposure), it may not keep up.

Worse, your gut might be reabsorbing old estrogen instead of helping eliminate it. And when those estrogen metabolites don't get cleared properly, they can recirculate, leading to **estrogen dominance**, even when your overall estrogen levels are technically low.

The result: mood swings, irritability, water retention, anxiety, and stubborn belly fat that won't budge. These are classic signs of hormonal imbalance that have less to do with how much estrogen you're producing and more to do with how well your body is clearing it.

Blood Sugar & Insulin Burden: The Hidden Drain on Detox

Think blood sugar only matters if you're diabetic? Think again.

Blood sugar swings are one of the *sneakiest* ways women in midlife overload their livers. Every spike and crash isn't just about energy dips or cravings; it's also a metabolic mess your liver has to clean up.

Here's what happens behind the scenes:

- When your blood sugar goes up, your pancreas pumps out insulin to bring it back down.
- That insulin surge tells your liver to get involved storing, converting, and clearing out the excess.
- Do that enough times (hello, stress snacking, skipped meals, or that second oat milk latte), and your liver is *constantly* on cleanup duty.

And it's not just about food. Stress, poor sleep, and hormone fluctuations can all spike your blood sugar, too, *even if you're eating clean.*

Midlife Makes You More Sensitive

Estrogen and Progesterone help keep insulin in check. So, when those hormones drop, your sensitivity to carbs and sugar shifts. Suddenly, the same foods you used to eat without issue are *causing* weight gain, inflammation, and blood sugar rollercoasters.

That "last ten pounds"? The constant three p.m. crash? The irritability or brain fog after meals? All signs your liver may be working overtime on sugar duty.

Where Things Start to Unravel

When insulin is always high, your liver gets bogged down. It loses capacity for the *other* important jobs, like clearing out excess hormones, toxins, and cholesterol. Over time, this can lead to insulin resistance (the precursor to prediabetes),[11] weight gain that won't budge, and metabolic dysfunction—that's when your body stops efficiently converting food into energy, and everything feels harder: sleep, mood, workouts, and focus.

The best part is that your body isn't malfunctioning; it just needs a different strategy.

And while hormones and blood sugar might be the loudest disruptors at first glance, there are deeper forces at play quietly draining your energy, clarity, and resilience.

When the systems we've just covered are under pressure, your body starts firing off warning signals. An overburdened liver doesn't just stall detox, it ripples out into other functions, creating symptoms that show up in surprising places. One of the biggest ripple effects is on your thyroid.

The Silent Saboteur: Thyroid Conversion & the Liver

You've checked your labs. Your doctor says your thyroid looks "normal." So why are you still dragging through your days, cold all the time, or gaining weight for no reason?

What's Really Going On

Most thyroid tests only look at TSH and maybe T4—but your *active* thyroid hormone is T3—and guess where that is made? That's right: your liver.

Here's how it works:

- Your thyroid gland produces mostly T4, the inactive form.

---

[11] "Insulin Resistance & Prediabetes," *National Institute of Diabetes and Digestive and Kidney Diseases,* https://www.niddk.nih.gov/health-information/diabetes/overview/what-is-diabetes/predia betes-insulin-resistance.

- Your liver (and a little bit of your gut) converts T4 into T3, the hormone your cells actually use.
- If your liver is overwhelmed, inflamed, or nutrient-deficient, this conversion slows down ... even if your thyroid gland itself is doing just fine.

Why Midlife Women Are at Risk

- Estrogen shifts can increase inflammation and impact the enzymes needed for conversion.
- Gut dysfunction (also common in midlife) can impair conversion too, especially if you're low in beneficial bacteria or struggling with nutrient absorption.
- And, a liver overloaded by meds, toxins, alcohol, or blood sugar spikes just doesn't have the bandwidth to handle it all.

Common Clues This Is Happening

These symptoms often get brushed off or misattributed, but if your T3 is low, you might notice:

- Fatigue that doesn't lift
- Brain fog or trouble focusing
- Feeling cold, especially hands and feet
- Dry skin or brittle nails
- Weight gain despite "doing everything right"
- Depression or low motivation
- Slowed digestion or constipation

Why This Matters

If your liver can't make enough T3, your metabolism slows to a crawl. And no amount of willpower, caffeine, or cardio will fix that. You need your conversion engine running smoothly—and that means giving your liver a break and addressing the hidden burdens holding it back.

Cholesterol & Fatty Liver: When "Clean Eating" Isn't Enough

If you've been told your cholesterol is "creeping up" or that you might have a fatty liver, even though you don't drink much and eat relatively well, you're in good company.

Midlife throws a double punch here: Your declining estrogen alters how your body manages fat and cholesterol, *and* your liver is already running a marathon trying to keep up with hormones, toxins, and inflammation. It's no wonder this system starts waving the white flag.

Let's break it down.

Cholesterol Shifts in Midlife

Estrogen plays a big role in cholesterol metabolism. When it starts to drop:

- LDL (often called the "bad" cholesterol) tends to rise
- HDL (the "good" one) might dip
- Triglycerides can start climbing, especially if blood sugar is swinging

Even if your diet hasn't changed, your body's response to fat has. That's why "normal" routines stop working. Your liver isn't processing and clearing cholesterol as efficiently anymore, and it shows up in your labs.

The Fatty Liver Dilemma

You don't have to be drinking margaritas or eating junk food to develop non-alcoholic fatty liver disease (NAFLD). Many women in midlife are being diagnosed with early signs of NAFLD despite eating clean, moving daily, and "doing everything right."

Why? Because of a sluggish, overwhelmed liver, meaning it:

- Can't keep up with blood sugar regulation
- Has trouble processing fats
- Struggles to clear out excess hormones and inflammatory byproducts

The result? Fat starts accumulating *in the liver itself.*

It's a vicious cycle: Fatty liver increases systemic inflammation → which impairs metabolism → which worsens blood sugar balance → which further burdens the liver.

Add in chronic stress and poor sleep, and you've got the perfect storm for metabolic slowdown, regardless of how clean you're eating.

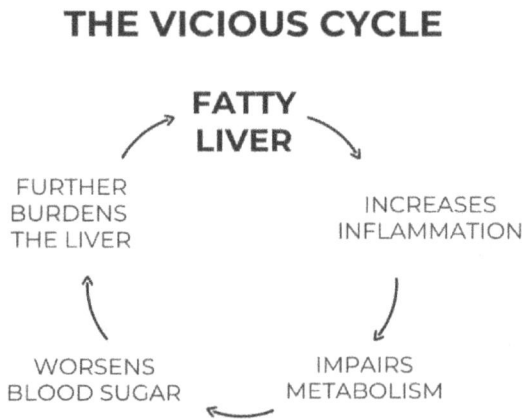

THE VICIOUS CYCLE

FATTY LIVER

FURTHER BURDENS THE LIVER

INCREASES INFLAMMATION

WORSENS BLOOD SUGAR

IMPAIRS METABOLISM

This isn't just theory. Let me show you what this looks like in real life.

When the Liver is the Missing Link

I once worked with a client in her late forties who ate clean, worked out daily, barely drank, and still couldn't shake her rising cholesterol, blood sugar swings, and stubborn weight gain.

Her doctor wanted to put her on statins. But when we tested her liver function and saw early signs of NAFLD, it became clear the issue wasn't fat intake. It was liver burden.

Once we focused on supporting her detox pathways and stabilizing blood sugar, everything started to shift: her labs improved, the weight came off, and—perhaps most importantly—she felt like herself again.

Why This Matters

When your liver is overburdened, everything else backs up:

- Hormones don't clear properly (hello, estrogen dominance)
- Detox pathways stall
- Inflammation ramps up
- Energy tanks
- Weight loss becomes *so much harder*

This is why supporting the liver isn't just "nice to have," it's non-negotiable in midlife. You'll learn how to support this powerhouse organ later in the book. But for now, just know: If your liver is struggling, your whole system feels it.

Next up, we're diving into the most overlooked signal your body is sending and how decoding your symptoms can change everything.

TL;DR—Chapter 3: Your Liver's Cry for Help—The Hidden Load You're Carrying

- Your liver is your body's multitasking powerhouse, managing detox, blood sugar, hormones, cholesterol, and thyroid conversion all at once.
- In midlife, the workload piles up from years of medications, birth control, food intolerances, alcohol, caffeine, and environmental toxins.
- Add in hormone fluctuations and blood sugar swings, and the liver gets clogged, slowing detox and creating ripple effects across your whole body.
- A sluggish liver leads to estrogen dominance, thyroid slowdown, high cholesterol, fatty liver, inflammation, stubborn weight, and bone-deep fatigue.
- Once you lower the hidden burden—by lightening the toxic load, supporting detox pathways, and stabilizing blood sugar—your liver can rebound, and your symptoms begin to shift.

Bottom line: If your liver is overloaded, everything else backs up. Supporting it isn't optional; it's the key to restoring energy, balance, and resilience in midlife.

Chapter 4: Your Body Is Talking. Are You Listening?

What if your symptoms weren't problems to fix ... but messages to decode?

That's the shift we're about to make.

You've seen how everything in midlife is connected: hormones, blood sugar, digestion, detox, and stress. Now let's zoom in. Because the fatigue, bloating, brain fog, mood swings, or stubborn weight you're feeling are not just frustrating symptoms, they're clues. But more than that, they're *data*—real information you can use.

In this chapter, we'll unpack what your body's trying to tell you one signal at a time so you can stop guessing and start taking action that actually works *for you.*

Reality Check: From Frustration to Curiosity

You wake up tired, even after eight hours of sleep. You eat clean and exercise regularly, but your jeans feel tighter by the week. You walk into a room and can't remember why. And then there's the bloating, the mood swings, the stubborn weight, and the fog that won't lift.

And at some point, the question hits you: *"Am I just supposed to accept this because I'm getting older?"*

It's a question I hear from almost every woman I work with. And it's usually followed by a string of frustrated thoughts:

- *I'm so tired of feeling tired.*
- *Why is my belly always bloated no matter what I eat?*
- *I must be losing my mind with this brain fog.*

- *My workouts aren't working anymore.*
- *I feel like a stranger in my own body.*

You've probably shared these concerns with someone, maybe even your doctor, and heard the standard midlife brush-off:

"Your labs look fine."

"It's just stress."

"That's normal for your age."

"Try eating less and moving more."

At first, you nod and go along with it. But deep down, it doesn't sit right. Because *you know something's off.*

And you're right.

This isn't you being lazy, dramatic, or overly sensitive. Your body isn't defective, and you're definitely not imagining things.

What if these symptoms aren't your enemy but your body waving a flag, asking for your attention?

Your body doesn't use words; it speaks in symptoms. And every one of those symptoms—no matter how small or strange—is a message.

They're your body's way of saying, *Hey, something's "off." Pay attention!*

When you start viewing symptoms as information (rather than annoyances), you shift from frustration to power, from helplessness to curiosity. So instead of asking yourself, *How do I make this go away?* You get to ask, *What is my body trying to tell me?* When you shift your mindset and stop seeing symptoms as something to silence, everything changes.

Symptoms = Your Body's Language

Think of your symptoms like a check engine light in your car. They're not proof that something is broken; they're simply a signal that something needs attention. You wouldn't just unplug the warning light to make it disappear; you'd investigate what triggered it. Your body works the same way. The goal isn't to silence the signal; it's to understand what it's pointing to.

That's where everything changes. And we're headed there next.

Ready to start listening differently?

To help you begin tracking these messages in real life (not just in theory), I created the **Body Talk Journal** as a bonus resource.

Inside, you'll find simple prompts and symptom tracking tools to help you spot patterns, notice what your body is asking for, and start making sense of what used to feel random.

☞ https://YourMidlifeBodyCode.com/bonuses

Now let's break it down symptom by symptom so you can start connecting the dots and crack *your* unique **Midlife Body Code**.

Let's start decoding.

Decoding the Signals

Once you start paying attention to your symptoms, you'll notice they're not random at all. They follow patterns. They show up in clusters. And they almost always point to a deeper root. Let's take a closer look at what your most common midlife symptoms might be trying to tell you.

Fatigue (All-Day or Afternoon Crash)

You wake up already tired, push through the day with coffee and willpower, and crash hard by three p.m., only to second-guess whether you've "done enough" to earn rest. Sound familiar? Fatigue is one of the most common (and most misunderstood) signals your body sends. It's not a lack of motivation; it's your internal systems struggling to meet your energy demands.

Here's what might be going on behind the scenes:

- **Mineral depletion**. Especially sodium, potassium, and magnesium. These key electrolytes power cellular energy. When they're low, your cells can't function optimally, and everything slows down.
- **Blood sugar instability**. Every crash after a carb-heavy lunch or a missed meal sends your body into emergency mode, draining reserves just to stabilize you.
- **Nervous system stuck in overdrive**. When you're constantly in fight-or-flight mode, your body prioritizes quick, short-term energy, not sustained fuel.
- **Liver and gut congestion**. If detox pathways are overloaded, waste builds up. That internal backlog can leave you feeling foggy, puffy, and sluggish.

What Your Body's Telling You: Your body isn't lazy; it's running on empty. The solution isn't more caffeine or pushing harder; it's rebuilding what your body has been burning through for years.

Stubborn Weight (Especially Belly Fat)

Despite doing "all the right things" (eating clean, working out, etc.), the scale won't budge. Or worse, it creeps up. And the weight that *does* show up? It's not just about how your clothes fit; it's about inflammation, puffiness, and the heavy, uncomfortable feeling that makes you feel disconnected from your body.

This isn't a willpower issue. It's not because you're doing something wrong. It's your body prioritizing survival over fat burning, and it's actually trying to *protect* you.

Here's what might be happening under the surface:

- **Insulin resistance**. When blood sugar is constantly spiking (from food, stress, or poor sleep), your cells stop responding to insulin. That keeps sugar circulating in your blood instead of being used for energy, and the excess gets stored as fat.
- **Elevated cortisol**. Chronically high stress hormones keep your body in a fat-storing, muscle-burning state. Cortisol tells your body to hold onto belly fat "just in case."
- **Gut and liver congestion.** Inflammation from food sensitivities, gut bugs, or sluggish detox slows down your metabolism and encourages the body to store fat as a protective buffer.

What Your Body's Telling You: Your body isn't sabotaging you; it's conserving resources and trying to stay safe. Fat storage is a survival response, not a failure. The real fix starts with lowering the internal burden so your body can shift out of defense mode.

Bloating & Digestive Discomfort

Some days, you feel fine. Other days, you're so bloated it's hard to button your jeans by three p.m. Or maybe you're gassy, burpy, constipated, dealing with loose stools—or all the above. It's uncomfortable, unpredictable, and often embarrassing. But digestive issues aren't just a nuisance; they're your gut's warning light.

This isn't about "too many vegetables" or eating too fast. It's about your digestive system being overloaded and under-supported.

Here's what might be going on behind the scenes:

- **Gut bugs and overgrowth**. When stomach acid or digestive enzymes are low, it's harder to break down food properly, which gives bacteria and yeast more fuel to ferment, leading to gas, bloating, and discomfort.
- **Food sensitivities**. Gluten, dairy, sugar alcohols, and other common irritants can trigger bloating, even if you've eaten them for years without issue.
- **Stress and nervous system dysregulation**. Digestion only works properly when your body feels safe. If your system is in fight-or-flight, stomach acid and enzymes don't get released and things don't move the way they should.

What Your Body's Telling You: Your gut isn't overreacting; it's overwhelmed. And every bloaty day is your body asking for more support, not more Tums.

Brain Fog & Mood Swings

You lose your train of thought mid-sentence. You forget simple words. You feel emotionally off, and sometimes you snap at people you love, then feel guilty an hour later. It's not just frustrating; it's disorienting, like your brain and emotions are no longer under your control. But brain fog and mood swings don't happen in a vacuum. They're deeply connected to what's going on inside your body.

Here's what might be driving them:

- **Blood sugar crashes**. When your blood sugar drops too low, your brain doesn't get the fuel it needs to function clearly. That's when the fog sets in and your fuse gets *really* short.
- **Mineral imbalances**. Minerals like sodium, potassium, and magnesium are the unsung heroes behind clear thoughts and steady moods. When they're running low, your brain is like a phone on five percent battery—foggy, glitchy, and way more likely to snap at someone.
- **Gut-brain connection**. Inflammation in your gut can create inflammation in your brain. And since your gut makes most of your feel-good neurotransmitters (like serotonin and dopamine), poor digestion can tank your focus and emotional resilience and even trigger anxiety and depression.

What Your Body's Telling You: You're not scattered or moody "for no reason." When your brain isn't getting the fuel, minerals, or gut support it needs, it *can't* think clearly or regulate your emotions. These aren't personality flaws; they're biochemical traffic jams. And they're absolutely fixable.

Still wondering if brain fog is "just part of aging"?

Brain fog is your brain on low fuel and low support. You're not losing your mind; you're losing access to nutrients, blood sugar stability, and calm. Don't ignore the fog. It's a sign that your body needs more support.

Why You're Snapping (Even When You Don't Mean To)

You promised yourself you'd stay calm. But then your partner says the *wrong* thing ... or your kid won't stop tapping ... or someone dares to breathe too loudly and too suddenly, and you're snapping. Again. And then comes the guilt: *Why did I lose it over something so small?*

But here's the truth: this isn't about being "too emotional" or needing more self-control. This is what happens when a nervous system has been on high alert for too long. You're not overreacting; you're overloaded. The irritability, the edginess, the feeling like your reactions are bigger than the moment— they're not character flaws—they're red flags from a body that's trying to keep up with everything you've been carrying.

Here's what could be pushing you to the edge:

- **Nervous system dysregulation**. When your body perceives ongoing demands as threats (even if they're not "big" ones), it shifts into survival mode. That means you're more reactive, easily overwhelmed, and constantly on alert because your body doesn't feel safe.
- **Blood sugar instability**. When your blood sugar drops, your brain panics. That can make you feel

impatient, jittery, snappy, or like you've suddenly gone from fine to frantic.

- **Hormone fluctuations**. In perimenopause, shifts in estrogen and progesterone can mess with the brain chemicals (GABA and serotonin) that keep you calm and centered. So even small triggers feel like *too much*.

What Your Body's Telling You: You're not crazy. You're just maxed out, and your body is calling for backup. When your nervous system is in overdrive and your blood sugar is crashing, even small stressors feel huge. This isn't about willpower, it's about overload. And when you lower the internal pressure, the reactivity melts away, too.

Apparently, Sleep Is Optional Now? (So Tired. So Awake.)

You crawl into bed exhausted, but your body is suddenly wide awake, replaying the day or worrying about something random, like whether you remembered to defrost the chicken. Or maybe you *do* fall asleep fast, only to wake up at three a.m., staring at the ceiling, your mind buzzing and your body stuck in high alert.

And somehow, you still get up and power through—because that's what you do. You tell yourself this is just part of midlife. That waking up exhausted is normal now. That maybe you just don't need as much sleep anymore. But here's the truth: Your body isn't fine with five broken hours of sleep. It's not adapting; it's compensating. And over time, that compensation comes at a cost.

Let's look at what might actually be keeping you up (or waking you up) at night:

- **Cortisol is moonlighting**. If your nervous system is in overdrive, your body thinks it needs to stay alert. That second wind at ten p.m. or the three a.m. "ping"? It's not random, it's your stress hormones hijacking your circadian rhythm like a boss who emails you "just one more thing" right as you're logging off.

- **Blood sugar crash = body alarm**. When your blood sugar dips too low in the middle of the night (thanks to a skimpy dinner, wine/sugar/carbs, or not enough protein), your body panics, releases cortisol, and boom! You're wide awake, staring at the ceiling.
- **Your liver's doing overtime**. Midlife equals more hormones to process, more toxins to clear, and a liver that's like *I'm gonna need some help here*. When it's overwhelmed, sleep becomes shallow or fragmented. You're technically asleep but not really resting.
- **You're low on chill minerals**. Magnesium and potassium are like the off switches for your nervous system. When they're depleted, your body has no idea it's supposed to be asleep. It's like trying to power down a laptop with forty-seven tabs open.
- **Your gut bugs are throwing a rave**. Certain bacteria, parasites, and yeast love the night shift. If they're overgrown, their party triggers inflammation and cortisol, leaving you wide awake while your microbiome is doing the Macarena.

What Your Body's Telling You: You're not just "a bad sleeper." You're not too old, too anxious, or too wired for rest. You're exhausted—and your body *still* doesn't feel safe enough to shut down.

When your stress hormones are running the show, your blood sugar is on a rollercoaster, and your mineral tank is empty, sleep becomes optional, and your body treats rest like a luxury it can't afford. The answer isn't melatonin or sleep hygiene tips (though those can help). It's about sending your body the signal that it's finally safe to exhale.

Real Life: Yolanda's Story—How Decoding the Patterns Changed Everything

"I feel like my body is rejecting everything I try to do for it."
- Yolanda, mid-fifties

That was the first thing Yolanda said to me. She wasn't being dramatic; she was desperate.

She had once been the rock for everyone else. The one who got things done, made the plans, kept it all together. But after years of mounting symptoms (chronic insomnia, anxiety, nausea, brain fog, nerve pain), her body no longer felt like her own.

By the time we met, she could barely eat once a day. Her body felt like it was rejecting everything she put in. Her sleep was erratic at best. She couldn't focus. And worst of all, she couldn't figure out why. She'd tried acupuncture, clean eating, nervous system work, even tinctures and teas. Nothing made a dent.

But here's what I want you to hear: **It wasn't that she hadn't tried; it's that nothing she tried was hitting the right target.**

From a conventional perspective, her symptoms looked random. Anxiety and brain fog? OK. But nausea, nerve pain, weight loss, and heat intolerance too? It didn't add up. Most doctors either brushed it off as anxiety or assumed it must be hormonal. But when we started looking at *patterns* instead of isolated problems, the story changed.

On paper, Yolanda was dealing with:

- A depleted nervous system that couldn't downshift into calm
- Gut inflammation that disrupted digestion, absorption, and immunity
- Poor hormone clearance from a sluggish liver

- A burned-out stress response stuck in overdrive
- And a history of mold exposure, childhood trauma, and nutrient deficiencies

Her labs confirmed what her body had been trying to say all along: this wasn't "just stress." This was overload. We started slowly: stabilizing her nervous system, supporting her digestion, bringing in protein, minerals, and safety—without triggering her already-sensitive system. Week by week, things began to shift.

The two a.m. panic jolts stopped.

The stabbing nerve pain softened.

The nausea calmed.

Her brain started coming back online. And most importantly, *she started coming back to herself.*

Yolanda didn't just get better. She reclaimed something more profound: her clarity, her calm, her voice. She started waking up with more energy, less pain, and a sense of possibility she hadn't felt in years. As she put it, "I didn't think I'd ever get back to this version of me (the one who could enjoy her mornings without panic or pain). But now I'm looking forward to the day again."

She learned that her symptoms weren't random, mysterious, or made-up. They were messages—*data*—her body's way of saying, *I need something different.*

And when we stopped chasing the symptoms and started decoding? *Everything changed.*

You Can Learn to Decode Your Body

This isn't about becoming a functional medicine expert or understanding lab markers. It's about something much simpler and much more powerful: learning to observe what's happening, decode the information, and respond with intention.

That nagging bloat? It's not just annoying, it's *data.*

That afternoon crash? *Data.*

The irritability that sneaks in before dinner? *More data.*

When you stop seeing symptoms as "bad" and start seeing them as data, everything shifts.

Data gives you *direction*. Without it, you're groping around in the dark, trying one thing after another, hoping something sticks. But when you *have* the data, you can make clear, confident decisions that move the needle.

You don't have to know everything. You just have to start listening. Because once you do, your body will start telling you exactly what it needs.

Here's What's Next

Now that you understand your symptoms are valuable clues and powerful data points, it's time to start exploring what's draining your energy and throwing your body out of sync.

Some energy drains are obvious, like poor sleep or skipped meals. But others are hidden in plain sight. In the next chapter, we'll expose the silent leaks stealing your fuel and how to plug them so your body can finally exhale.

TL;DR – Chapter 4: Your Body Is Talking. Are You Listening?

- The symptoms you're facing in midlife—fatigue, bloating, brain fog, stubborn weight, mood swings—aren't random; they're your body's way of signaling imbalance.
- Symptoms are your body's language, like a check engine light: they're not proof something is broken, but clues about what needs attention.
- These signals often cluster together and point to underlying issues like blood sugar swings, mineral depletion, gut imbalances, hormone shifts, or a nervous system in overdrive.

- When you connect the dots and look at patterns instead of isolated complaints, you move from guessing to understanding what your body is really asking for.

Bottom line: Your body isn't broken; it's communicating. The more you listen, the easier it gets to give it what it truly needs.

Chapter 5: Why Generic Fixes Don't Work for You

Is This You?

You've done the Whole30.

You've tried keto, intermittent fasting, "clean eating."

You've joined the bootcamps, counted the macros, drank the green juices.

And yet ...

You're still tired.

Still inflamed.

Still stuck.

You followed the rules. You did the "right" things. So why do you still feel like crap? Do you find yourself thinking, *"What is wrong with me?"* Then this chapter is for you.

The Truth: Generic Fixes Don't Fix Unique Problems

Here's the truth most wellness plans won't tell you: Your body is not a one-size-fits-all machine.

What worked for your best friend ...

Or your favorite influencer ...

Or even your younger self ...

may not work for the woman you are now because your current needs aren't just based on willpower or calories.

They're shaped by:

- Your **mineral status** (Are your cells able to do their jobs?)

- Your **gut function and digestion** (Can you break down and absorb what you eat?)
- Your **hormone shifts** (Aren't perimenopause and menopause "fun"?)
- Your **liver detox capacity** (Can your body process what it's exposed to?)
- Your **nervous system regulation** (Are you stuck in "go" mode or able to recharge?)

It's not guesswork. These are real variables we can track, support, and shift.

And that's just the beginning.

Think of it like borrowing someone else's prescription glasses.

Maybe they *kind of* work. But over time, they leave you feeling worse—headaches, blurred vision, frustration. Because they weren't made for you. Generic health plans do the same thing. They give you someone else's prescription, without understanding your body's unique vision.

The Bioindividuality Picture

That's where bioindividuality comes in. Simply put, it's *your body, your blueprint*. No one else has your exact wiring. Bioindividuality means no two bodies process food, stress, or toxins the same way. Not even close.

I once had a client who drank twenty cups of coffee a day—yes, *twenty*. Not because she was trying to win some sort of caffeine contest, but because she regularly pulled all-nighters and somehow *functioned* the next day.

Most people would have ended up in the ER. She just kept going. It wasn't until much later that we discovered why her body handled it so differently: She had four kidneys. (Yes, really.)

Now, I don't recommend trying that at home, but it's a perfect example of how wildly different our bodies can be behind the scenes. This is why chasing the next health trend keeps letting you down. You're not doing it wrong; you're just following someone else's instructions for a completely different body.

That's why, later in this book, we'll get into the functional lab testing that helped so many of my clients uncover what was truly going on beneath the surface. But even without labs, tuning in to how your body responds is where personalization begins.

To help you start identifying what makes *you* unique—and why generic advice hasn't worked. I created a simple tool called **Your Personal Body Blueprint.**

(Grab it here, https://YourMidlifeBodyCode.com/bonuses.)

Think of it as a snapshot of what your body is navigating right now. The more you understand this, the clearer your next steps become.

From Guessing to Strategy: What Your Body's Trying to Tell You

You don't need to overhaul your life. You need to start noticing what your body is already telling you.

And the more data you gather—from your energy, sleep, mood, and digestion—the more empowered you are to take *specific*, supportive action.

That's the opposite of guessing. That's strategy. That's personalization.

Why Personalization is Freedom (Not Restriction)

Here is something most wellness advice gets completely backward: Personalization isn't about adding more to your plate. It's about finally being able to take things *off*.

When you know what your body needs, you can stop wasting time on:

- Programs that aren't designed for midlife women
- Workouts that spike your cortisol instead of building strength
- Diets that drain your energy and mess with your mood
- Supplements that promise everything but deliver nothing

The *truth* is that trying to do "all the things" is what has been making you feel like a failure.

But once you understand your body's unique code, you stop chasing trends and start getting traction. You make decisions that fit your physiology, not someone else's opinion. You start to see results. Not because you pushed harder, but because you supported your body smarter.

That's freedom.

Freedom from second-guessing.

Freedom from overwhelm.

Freedom from constantly trying to fix what's not actually broken, just misunderstood.

When you understand your code, you can finally support your body with clarity, not chaos.

What Personalization Looks Like (In Real Life)

Personalization comes alive when you see it in action. Here's how listening to your unique body signals and making targeted changes transformed real clients' health and energy:

- **One client came to me convinced she just needed to "try harder."** But once we tracked her symptoms, we saw a clear midday crash, bloating after certain meals, and poor sleep after workouts. Those patterns were data. We adjusted her food timing, added mineral support, and simplified her workouts. Her energy shot up— without doing *more*.

- **Beverly spent years being misdiagnosed with bladder infections.** The antibiotics never helped, and the flares kept coming, usually after sex or during high-stress seasons. Eventually, we connected the dots: mold exposure had triggered oxalate dumping, and those sharp crystals were irritating her bladder lining. No amount of cranberry juice or antibiotics could fix that. What helped? Reducing her toxic burden, calming her nervous system, and addressing the true root. The flares stopped when we started listening.

- **Kristy had done every elimination diet in the book.** No gluten, no dairy, no nightshades, yet *still*, the bloating and nausea stuck around. She couldn't tolerate most proteins or fats, and even "healthy" foods like onions or garlic left her doubled over. What we uncovered was a sluggish liver and poor bile flow, which made it nearly impossible for her to digest food properly. Once we supported her liver, things shifted fast: Her meals no longer triggered pain, and her energy started coming back online.

- **Another client felt completely dismissed by doctors who told her everything looked "normal."** But she wasn't fine. She was in pain, couldn't sleep, and her weight wouldn't budge, no matter what she tried. We took one look at her food and saw the problem: Her blood sugar was all over the place. She was starting her day with carbs, not getting enough protein, and crashing hard by afternoon. We adjusted her meals, gave her gut some support, and introduced simple tools to release stress and calm anxiety. She started sleeping through the night, her pain disappeared, and the weight finally started coming off—without trying harder, just differently.

- **Dana never left home without knowing where the nearest bathroom was.** She'd dealt with loose stools, bloating, and "food reactions" for years and carried an extra change of clothes in her purse, just in case. The real culprit? A gut overrun with pathogens that were disrupting digestion and driving inflammation. Once we gave her gut the targeted support it needed, the urgency and food issues finally eased. She felt safe in her body again, for the first time in years.

- **Maya had been told her thyroid was fine, despite dragging energy and cycling between anxiety and exhaustion.** But her symptoms kept stacking up: cold hands and feet, brittle nails, dry skin, and unpredictable periods. Eventually, functional testing confirmed what we already suspected: Hashimoto's, an autoimmune thyroid condition. But it wasn't the labs that saved her; it was the fact that she noticed the pattern and trusted her intuition when traditional answers fell short.

When you know how to read your body's signals, everything changes.

You stop blaming yourself and start doing what actually works. Now that you've started identifying the patterns in your body, it's time to stop following advice that was never designed for you and start responding with what your body needs.

In the next section, we'll begin the process of realigning. This is where the fog starts to lift. We'll walk through the biggest systems that need your support, starting with the ones draining your energy the most, and how to bring them back into balance.

TL;DR – Chapter 5: Why Generic Fixes Don't Work for You

- Generic diets, programs, and "one-size-fits-all" fixes don't work because they ignore your unique biology.
- Bioindividuality means your body has its own unique code. What works for others may backfire for you.
- Paying attention to your patterns—energy, mood, digestion, sleep—is the first step toward real answers.
- Personalization isn't about doing more; it's about doing what actually works for *you*.

Bottom line: Stop guessing, start observing. Your body already knows what it needs. You just have to learn how to read the signs.

Part 2: Realign

By now, you've started to connect the dots. You know your symptoms aren't random; they're data. You've seen how stress, inflammation, blood sugar swings, and gut issues can throw everything out of whack.

So ... now what?

In this section, we shift from decoding to doing. You'll learn how to realign your systems so your body can finally stop fighting itself and start working *with* you.

We're talking blood sugar, digestion, minerals, nervous system, and more. But not in a "fix everything overnight" way. This is about smart, strategic shifts that meet your body where it's at, today.

Because when you give your body what it actually needs—not what a 25-year-old influencer needs—everything changes.

Chapter 6: Energy Leaks & What's Really Draining You

Plugging hidden leaks is the fastest way to refill your tank.

You got a full night's sleep but still wake up tired. By two p.m., you're dragging. You try more coffee, another green juice, a power nap, but nothing really works. It feels like your body just doesn't *hold* energy anymore.

Here's why:

It's not a willpower problem.

It's not a sleep problem.

It's a **leak** problem.

Imagine trying to fill a bathtub with the drain wide open. That's what your body is doing: trying to generate energy while it's leaking out through hidden imbalances like blood sugar crashes, mineral depletion, and a nervous system stuck in overdrive.

This kind of exhaustion has been normalized, especially for high-achieving women like you. But just because it's common doesn't mean it's normal. And it definitely isn't because you're not "trying hard enough." Your body isn't failing; it's compensating, and doing its best with a foundation that's been drained.

Let's start plugging the leaks.

Where Your Energy's Really Going

Plugging the leaks starts with identifying them. And most of them aren't obvious.

This isn't just about skipping sleep or forgetting lunch. It's about the subtle, chronic imbalances that quietly drain your system all day long. These leaks don't always show up on standard labs, but your body feels them, especially in midlife, when your internal load is higher and your margins are thinner.

Your body *wants* to give you energy. But when the systems responsible for making, using, and conserving it are out of sync, that energy either doesn't show up or it disappears fast. This isn't a motivation problem; it's your body doing triage.

And for most women in this phase of life, energy isn't leaking from just one place. It's a combination of:

- **Low minerals** that make it harder for nutrients—and energy—to get into your cells
- **Blood sugar crashes** that pull the rug out from under you
- **A nervous system stuck in overdrive**, keeping you wired but never restored
- **A digestive system** that isn't breaking down or absorbing what you need
- **A sluggish liver** that's overworked and under-supported

These may sound like separate issues, but they all have one thing in common: **They burn through energy faster than you can replace it.**

If your body feels like it's running on fumes—even when you *should* feel rested—it's time to stop blaming your age, your schedule, or your willpower.

It's not about working harder. It's about giving your body the support it's been missing.

Let's break down the most common energy leaks and what you can do to start sealing them.

The Big Three Energy Leaks + Actionable Tips

Mineral Depletion—What Happens When the Tugboats Go on Strike?

If you're doing all the "right" things—sleeping, eating clean, working out, taking supplements—but still feel like a worn-out rag doll most days, you're not alone. And you're definitely not doing it wrong. You're just missing the key ingredient most midlife women overlook: minerals.

Some people call them the "spark plugs" of the body because they ignite almost every system, but I like to think of minerals as the little tugboats in a busy port. We need all the big cargo ships, like hormones, nutrients, and oxygen, coming in and out. But without the tugboats, those ships can't dock. They circle the harbor, going nowhere. And just like that jammed-up port, your body slows down. Everything backs up. Nothing gets delivered where it's needed.

These mineral "tugboats" don't get a lot of attention, but they're involved in nearly every function in the body. Without them, your cells literally can't make energy. That's why this is one of the first things I look at with clients. Because, if we don't fix this piece, it doesn't matter how great your workouts or supplements are, your body simply doesn't have what it needs to function.

What Minerals Actually Do

Magnesium alone is involved in over five hundred enzymatic reactions in the body, and it's one of the first things to tank when you're stressed (which, let's face it, is daily life for most of us). Sodium, potassium, and calcium round out what I call the "Big Four," and together they support everything from hydration to digestion to nervous system regulation.

I use this example with clients all the time: Imagine Mom goes on vacation for a week. When she gets home, the dishes are piled high, no one's eaten a real meal, and the laundry's a mess. That's what your body feels like when minerals are depleted. Everything gets backed up. Nothing runs smoothly. And you're left feeling foggy, frazzled, and flat-out exhausted.

Why You're Likely Depleted

There are a few reasons this is so common, especially in midlife.

First, stress burns through minerals like wildfire. Every time your body activates the stress response, it uses up potassium and magnesium. The longer you stay in that fight-or-flight state, the more depleted you become.

Second, our food isn't as rich in minerals as it used to be. Thanks to modern farming practices, our soil is depleted, and that means your spinach isn't packing the same punch it did fifty years ago.

And finally, a lot of women in this phase of life are unintentionally under-fueling. They see the weight creeping up, panic, and start eating less. But when your body is already running on empty, cutting calories just pushes you further into depletion. You can't fix a drained system by starving it.

Why It Matters: The Cell Battery Analogy

Every single cell in your body has a sodium-potassium pump—a little "see-saw" mechanism that controls what gets in and what gets out. Nutrients in, waste out. But if those minerals are off, the pump doesn't work. It's like trying to charge your phone with a frayed cord. Nothing connects. Nothing holds.

That's why you might be doing all the right things and still feel like garbage. The fuel is there, but it's not getting where it needs to go.

Of course, testing can give us valuable insight, but you don't have to wait for lab results to start making changes. Supporting your minerals with nutrient-dense food, hydration, and smart supplementation can help you feel better now. The testing just helps us fine-tune.

What I See on HTMA Tests

When I run hair tissue mineral analysis (HTMA) with clients, here's what I see again and again: low sodium, low potassium, low magnesium. Your key minerals are wiped out. And, without them, your body is trying to run a race with no gas in the tank.

Some women also show a calcium shell pattern, whereby calcium is leached out of the bones and teeth (where we want it) to buffer stress in the body. If this goes on too long, however, it ends up slowing your metabolism, thyroid, and detox pathways. It can feel like you're walking through wet cement: heavy, sluggish, and stuck. And in some women, it can be even more detrimental: Excreted calcium can pool in the body, showing up as joint pain, gallstones, kidney stones, calcification of the arteries, or even frozen shoulder.

And then there's copper. Most women don't know they're dealing with copper toxicity until the symptoms start stacking up: mood swings, estrogen dominance, insomnia, anxiety, even hair loss. If you've ever been on birth control or had a copper IUD, it's worth exploring. Copper sits on the brain and is often referred to as an "emotional mineral." In the wrong amount, it can mess with your mood in a way that makes you question your sanity.

What About Hair Loss?

If your ponytail is thinning or you notice more hair in the shower drain, you are not imagining it, and you are not alone. Hair loss in midlife is incredibly common, and it is rarely just about "aging."

- **Minerals matter.** Low sodium, potassium, and magnesium (all common on HTMA) mean your cells cannot make energy or move nutrients where they need to go. Copper toxicity, in particular, can throw off thyroid function and drive hair shedding.
- **Thyroid connection.** Your thyroid is like your body's thermostat, and when minerals are out of balance, that thermostat goes haywire. One of the first places it shows is in your hair.
- **Fueling counts.** If you are under-eating (a common reaction when weight creeps up in midlife), your body will prioritize survival over hair growth.

Once we correct the mineral imbalances, support thyroid function, and ensure you are eating enough, your hair often begins to rebound. It takes time (because hair cycles run in months, not days), but regrowth is possible.

How to Start Rebuilding

You don't need a complete overhaul to start feeling better. You need a few key shifts to support mineral balance and energy production:

- **Eat enough.** This is non-negotiable. If you're trying to heal on twelve hundred calories a day, it's not going to work. Most midlife women need at least fifteen hundred to two thousand calories/day, depending on height and metabolic needs.
- **Protein and healthy fats.** Aim for twenty to thirty grams of protein at each meal. Not only does this support muscle and blood sugar, but protein also delivers key amino acids and minerals that fuel repair.
- **Adrenal cocktails.** These help replenish sodium and potassium, two minerals that crash under chronic stress. I customize these based on your HTMA results, but popular options include coconut water or cream of tartar, sea salt, and freshly squeezed lemon juice.
- **Magnesium baths or topicals.** If digestion is sluggish, skip the pills, and try Epsom salt baths or magnesium lotion. Your skin is a great absorption pathway, especially when your gut isn't cooperating.
- **Rethink vitamin D.** If you're a slow oxidizer (which many women are), too much vitamin D can actually drag down your energy and metabolism. If you're already supplementing and not feeling better (or feeling worse), it may be worth reevaluating. This is where personalized testing helps fine-tune your approach.

Your Next Step

Want to know exactly how to support your mineral balance based on your own patterns?

Scan the QR code below or visit https://YourMidlife BodyCode.com/bonuses to download your **Mineral Support Guide**. Inside, you'll find food ideas, supplement strategies, adrenal cocktail recipes, and more tips to start boosting energy the smart way.

Blood Sugar Rollercoaster: The Invisible Drain

If your energy feels like it tanks out of nowhere—one minute you're fine, and the next you're snapping at someone or trying not to fall asleep at your desk—there's a good chance your blood sugar is to blame.

And no, I'm not talking about diabetes. I'm talking about the daily swings most women don't realize they're stuck in. You skip breakfast, chug a latte, rush into your day, maybe grab a protein bar or a cheese stick around one p.m., and by dinnertime, you're ravenous. So, you overeat (or eat too fast) and feel bloated, heavy, and foggy the rest of the night. Sound familiar?

Those ups and downs are what I call the blood sugar rollercoaster. And in midlife, it's not just annoying, it's *exhausting*. You feel good after eating, then crash. You're clear-headed in the morning, then you can't focus by two p.m. You get hangry between meals, are wired at three a.m., and too tired to work out but too restless to rest. And the longer that ride continues, the more it impacts your inflammation, hormones, weight, sleep, and mood. It's one of the most overlooked (and most fixable) energy drains I see.

Symptoms of Blood Sugar Swings

Before your labs ever flag a problem, symptoms often show up in two distinct ways:

- **Low blood sugar**—when your blood sugar dips between meals or overnight
- **Insulin resistance**—when your body struggles to process sugar, even if labs still look "normal"

When Blood Sugar Drops, Symptoms Include:

- Feeling "hangry" if you go too long without eating
- Spacey, light-headed, or shaky between meals
- Energy spikes (and crashes) right after eating
- No appetite in the morning or waking up slightly nauseated
- Big afternoon energy dips or needing a nap to push through
- Waking up at three or four a.m. full of energy
- Brain fog or trouble concentrating between meals

When Insulin Can't Keep Up, Symptoms Include:

- Feeling tired after meals
- Sugar cravings after eating
- Trouble losing weight (despite doing "everything right")
- Waist larger than hips
- Frequent urination or feeling hungry again too soon

These signs may show up long before your glucose is "abnormal" on blood labs. That's why fasting insulin and other markers are better early indicators.

Blood Sugar and Energy

Think of these swings like sprinting and collapsing all day long. Your body surges to keep you going, then drops hard when that burst runs out. That rollercoaster depletes your minerals, spikes cortisol, worsens cravings, and increases inflammation. Here's what changes everything: *Stabilizing your blood sugar is one of the fastest ways to feel steadier, calmer, and energized, without needing to overhaul your entire life.*

What Works to Stabilize Blood Sugar

Before we get into the specifics, here are two foundational pieces to remember:

- **Stick to real, whole foods as often as possible.** Your body doesn't just need calories; it needs nutrients. Processed foods, even the "healthy" kind, often lack the protein, fat, and fiber your body needs to stay steady.
- **Give your system a rest.** Aim for twelve to fourteen hours between dinner and breakfast (like seven p.m. to seven to nine a.m.). This gentle fasting window supports insulin sensitivity and gives your digestion time to reset without stressing your system like longer fasts can.

Here are some of the shifts I recommend most:

- **Prioritize protein.** Twenty to thirty grams per meal (especially breakfast). It builds muscle, keeps you full, and helps prevent the mid-afternoon crash.
- **Balance your snacks.** If you're eating enough at meals (especially getting twenty to thirty grams of protein), you

shouldn't *need* to snack. But, if you're still rebuilding your metabolism, a smart snack can help. Just skip the lone apple or granola bar. Pair carbs with protein, fat, or fiber to stay steady: a hard-boiled egg and a few olives, hummus and veggies, almonds and turkey. Fruit is fine, just don't eat it solo. Always pair it with a protein or healthy fat.

- **Don't fear carbs, just pair them wisely.** Instead of going no-carb, focus on combining your carbs with fat, protein, or fiber. That slows the spike and gives you lasting fuel.
- **Eat enough.** Under-eating (especially during the day) leads to over-eating or cravings at night. And if you're constantly under-fueling, your blood sugar and cortisol will pay the price.
- **Try a continuous glucose monitor (CGM) or glucometer.** These tools help you spot what foods or habits cause spikes and crashes. If you love data, this can be eye-opening, but you don't *need* one to start seeing benefits.

Tips from the Glucose Revolution

- Add a green starter (like a salad) before your main dish

Jessie Inchauspé's work on blood sugar has helped bring this conversation into the mainstream.[12] Here are a few of her simple, science-backed hacks:

- Eat your meals in this order for better blood sugar balance: veggies → protein → carbs
- Drink 1 tbsp. of apple cider vinegar in water before meals

---

[12] Jessie Inchauspé, *Glucose Revolution: The Life-Changing Power of Balancing Your Blood Sugar*, (Simon Element, 2022).

- Move your body within sixty minutes of eating (walk, stretch, squats, calf raises—whatever works!)
- If you're going to have sugar, eat it *after* a meal, not as a snack

These small changes help flatten the spikes, lower inflammation, and give you steadier energy all day long.

Why Midlife Isn't the Time to Fast Hard

In your twenties, intermittent fasting might've felt like a great reset. But in midlife, especially with shifting hormones and blood sugar swings, it can actually backfire.

When your adrenals and metabolism are already under pressure, skipping meals drives cortisol higher, slows metabolism, and increases insulin resistance.

The smarter move? *Fuel your body intentionally and* consistently in a way that supports your energy, not drains it.

Nervous System Overdrive: The Energy Thief

When your nervous system is stuck in overdrive, even rest doesn't feel restorative.

Your mind might be telling you it's time to relax, but if your body is still operating in a state of hypervigilance—tense muscles, shallow breathing, heart racing—you'll stay locked in "go" mode whether you like it or not. This constant low-level stress response burns through your energy reserves, leaving you tired, irritable, and unable to recharge.

If you're feeling wired but tired, struggling to fall asleep, waking in the middle of the night, or snapping at the people you love over minor things, your nervous system might be stuck in fight-or-flight. And when that happens, your body prioritizes survival over everything else, including digestion, hormone production, and deep repair.

This isn't just about stress in the way most people think of it (mental and emotional overwhelm). Physical and biochemical stressors like pain, inflammation, gut bugs, mold, or blood sugar swings also contribute to nervous system overload and elevated cortisol.

Over time, this constant activation can lead to adrenal fatigue, poor resilience, and a deep sense of burnout. Here's the best part: The fix doesn't have to be complex. It's about building in what I call Daily Downshifts—simple, short practices that signal to your body that it's safe to power down.

Daily Downshifts to Calm the System

Here are some of my favorite nervous system reset tools— think of these as your personal "calm buffet." **Take what works, leave what doesn't**, and *start with just one or two* if you feel overwhelmed.

Breathwork

Just three deep breaths can tell your brain, *We're safe now.* Try this:

- Inhale for four counts
- Hold for two counts
- Exhale slowly for six to eight counts

Repeat three times. This longer exhale activates your parasympathetic nervous system, your rest-and-digest mode.

Tapping (EFT)

Tap through acupressure points to calm the brain and body. It may feel odd at first, but studies show EFT (Emotional Freedom Technique) reduces anxiety, depression, PTSD, and even food cravings.

Adaptogens

These powerful herbs help buffer the effects of chronic stress. Favorites include ashwagandha, rhodiola, holy basil, and maca. I often add powdered versions to smoothies or teas.

Essential Oils

Aromatherapy works. Try lavender for sleep, frankincense for pain and inflammation, or lemon for an uplifting midday reset.

Movement

Movement helps complete the stress cycle and release lingering tension. Walking, gentle yoga, stretching, and even a solo dance party can help your body reset.

Legs Up the Wall

Lie down, put your legs up the wall for five to ten minutes. This calming pose helps improve circulation and calms the vagus nerve.

Magnesium & Mineral Baths

Stress drains your mineral reserves, especially magnesium, which plays a key role in calming the nervous system. Epsom salt or magnesium chloride baths can replenish your stores *and* help your body shift out of fight-or-flight. Try adding one to two cups of Epsom salt or magnesium flakes to warm water and soak for twenty minutes.

Tech Breaks

Even five minutes of screen-free time—just you and the trees, a cup of tea, or a few deep breaths—can help bring your nervous system back online.

Building a Practice That Works for You

The key here isn't doing everything; it's doing something consistently. Calming your nervous system is like building a new muscle. The more you practice, the stronger your baseline becomes. These small, consistent shifts help send your body the message it's been waiting for: *You're safe now.* And once your nervous system truly feels safe, that's when the real repair work can begin.

Gut & Liver Load: The Hidden Energy Drain

Before we move on, there are two more major energy thieves worth mentioning: your gut and liver. If your digestion is sluggish or your liver is overloaded, your body has to work overtime just to keep up with the basics, leaving less energy for *you*. Think of it this way: If your body is constantly managing gut inflammation or trying to clear out a backlog of toxins, it's like running a full-time cleanup crew behind the scenes. No wonder you feel depleted.

You'll dive deeper into these issues in the next chapter, *The Puffy, Bloated, Inflamed Body*, but just know: Your energy isn't just about sleep, food, or mindset. It's also about what your body is silently battling on the inside.

Client Case Study: Plugging the Leaks

Remember Janice from Chapter 1? When we first met, she was frustrated, foggy, and flat-out exhausted. She kept pushing harder (trying stricter diets, longer workouts, and more supplements), thinking that if she just did everything *perfectly*, her energy would come back.

What she didn't realize was that her exhaustion wasn't from doing too little; it was from running on empty. Her hair mineral test showed significant mineral depletion (especially sodium and potassium), and her food journal revealed a pattern I see all the time: skipping meals, under-eating during the day, then trying to "be good" by avoiding snacks at night ... only to end up binging or crashing. She was also stuck in chronic nervous system overdrive. Even when she rested, her body didn't. She described it as being "tired but wired," like she was never fully off.

Instead of throwing more at her, we simplified by adding adrenal cocktails and strategic mineral support. She started eating balanced meals with enough protein *consistently* and worked in short Daily Downshifts, like breathing practices and stepping away from tech throughout her day. In just a few weeks, her afternoon crashes decreased, her sleep improved, and her energy started to feel more stable.

No crash diets. No overhauls. Just targeted tweaks based on her unique body.

Stop Trying Harder—Start Sealing the Leaks

If there's one thing I want you to take from this chapter, it's this:

You don't need to "push through"—you need to *seal the leaks*.

Back in Chapter 2, I told you you're not broken. Now you're starting to see why. You've been running a high-performance machine without fuel, and it's time to change that. You're working with a depleted foundation. And no amount of willpower can override a nervous system stuck in overdrive, a body starved for minerals, or blood sugar swinging like a pendulum.

This isn't about doing more. It's about supporting the right systems so your body can finally do what it's designed to do: function, thrive, and restore.

Energy is the first domino. When you fix this, everything else starts getting easier—your focus, your mood, your motivation, even your ability to work out or plan meals. But this only happens when you stop draining your tank. Once that tank starts to refill, you can battle the puffiness, bloating, and inflammation that's been making you feel "off" in your own body. And that's where we're headed next.

TL;DR – Chapter 6: Energy Leaks & What's Really Draining You

- Midlife exhaustion isn't a willpower problem; it's energy leaking out through hidden drains.
- The biggest culprits are mineral depletion (low sodium, potassium, magnesium), blood sugar swings, and a nervous system stuck in overdrive.
- A sluggish gut and liver add to the burden, silently draining your reserves.
- These leaks burn through energy faster than you can replace it, leaving you wired, tired, or both.
- Sealing the leaks doesn't require an overhaul, just steady, supportive shifts that refill your tank.

Bottom line: You're not failing, you're leaking. Plug the drains, and your energy becomes the first domino that helps everything else fall back into place.

Chapter 7: The Puffy, Bloated, Inflamed Puzzle

It's not fat; it's fluid. Your body is protecting you.

You wake up and your rings are tight, and your ankles are swollen. Your stomach is flat(ish) in the morning, but by noon, your jeans are cutting into your waist, and your bra band feels like a tourniquet. You catch a glimpse of your reflection and think, *Why am I so puffy*? You didn't eat a loaf of bread in your sleep, so what gives?

This isn't about "just getting older." And it's not that you've "let yourself go." You cut back on carbs. You're exercising. You're eating *healthier than ever*. And yet ... the puff persists.

For some women, the swelling is visible on their face. For others, it shows up in their hands, fingers, ankles, and waistline. My client, Lorena, told me, "I'm feeling so much less inflamed—my rings are loose! Stomach feels flat and not so bloated." (We'll hear more about her story in a few pages.)

Dana had been wearing her wedding ring on her pinkie for months, refusing to resize it out of sheer frustration. A few weeks into her protocol, she slipped it back onto her ring finger for the first time since she started and zipped up a coat she hadn't worn in years.

What you and my clients are feeling is a combination of two things: bloating and inflammation. They're different, but they often show up at the same time, making you feel heavy, puffy, uncomfortable, and frustrated.

Let's break down the difference:

- **Bloating** is what happens when gas gets trapped or digestion slows down. It's often driven by gut imbalances, food sensitivities, or poor enzyme function. It tends to fluctuate throughout the day, often better in the morning and worse after meals.
- **Inflammation**, on the other hand, is more systemic. It shows up as water retention, puffiness, skin issues, or a general feeling of "being inflamed" from the inside out. It's your immune system's response to overload, whether from toxins, gut bugs, hormone imbalances, or hidden food triggers.

Think of it this way: Bloating is in your belly. Inflammation is in your cells.

Both are your body asking for help. The encouraging part is that they're both addressable. You just need to understand what's driving them, and that's exactly what we're about to uncover.

Your Body's Inflammatory Load

This isn't just about what you eat. Your body is constantly juggling inputs, from gut bugs and food sensitivities to toxins, hormone imbalances, and stress. All of it adds to your inflammatory load, the total burden your body is carrying at any given time. And when that load gets too high, your body reacts by holding on to water to protect you. It's not fat. It's not failure. It's fluid—your body's way of protecting you from the internal stress it's under.

Understanding your inflammatory load is the key to feeling clear, light, and comfortable in your body again. So, let's look at what's driving it.

Top Signs It's Inflammation, Not Just Weight

- Your face looks puffier than usual, especially in the morning
- Your rings or shoes feel tight by midday
- You feel heavier, but the scale hasn't changed much
- Your joints or fingers feel swollen, even without injury
- You "deflate" a bit overnight, but puff back up by afternoon
- Your body feels squishy or watery, not solid
- You feel uncomfortable in clothes that *should* fit

These are signs your body is holding onto fluid—not fat—due to internal inflammation or overload.

The Root Causes of Puff, Bloat, and Inflammation

By now, you know this isn't just about eating too much or aging. That puffy/inflamed feeling is your body's response to overload. And it's usually not coming from just one place.

The three biggest contributors I see in midlife women are gut-health imbalances, liver overload, and hidden food triggers

1. Gut Health Imbalances

Your gut isn't just a digestion center; it's home to trillions of bacteria that impact your mood, immunity, and inflammation levels. When that ecosystem is out of balance, symptoms show up fast.

Common drivers:

- **Low stomach acid** or insufficient enzymes → poor breakdown of food
- **Gut bug overgrowth** (yeast, bacteria, parasites) → fermentation, trapped gas, and bloat
- **Leaky gut and food sensitivities** → immune response that shows up as puffiness, fatigue, or that "inflamed" feeling

When your gut is off, the microbes that should be helping you thrive end up getting pushed out by the ones causing gas, bloat, and inflammation.

Typical symptoms include:

- Bloating after meals
- Constipation, loose stools, or that "never fully emptied" feeling
- Excess gas or uncomfortable pressure that makes you unbutton your pants by three p.m.

You might be eating all the "right" foods, but if your gut can't digest and absorb them properly, you're not getting the benefits. And when food isn't properly broken down, your body may treat it like an intruder, not fuel.

2. Liver Overload

As discussed in previous chapters, our liver filters toxins, clears out old hormones, and helps eliminate what your body doesn't need. But when it's backed up, everything else slows down, including digestion, hormone clearance, and detox.

Common contributors:

- Alcohol (even a few glasses a week)
- Medications and over-the-counter painkillers
- Processed foods or chemical additives
- Too many supplements (yes, even the "healthy" ones)

Listen, no amount of green juice can unclog that "sink" if you're still downing wine, ibuprofen, and that cinnamon bun candle on the daily. It's unfair, I know. But you will feel *so* much better when you're not feeling the weight of a thousand toxins raining down on your system.

What it looks like when the liver is overburdened:

- Puffy face and water retention
- Skin issues, like breakouts or dullness
- Hormonal symptoms (PMS, acne, weight shifts)
- Headaches or sluggish digestion

You don't need another "cleanse," you need to reduce the burden so your liver can catch up.

3. Hidden Food Triggers

Sometimes it's not *what* you're eating but what your body can't tolerate *right now*. Inflammation makes your gut lining more permeable (like a sieve), which means even "healthy" foods can cause reactions until your system is more resilient.

The most common culprits?

- Gluten
- Dairy
- Refined sugar
- Alcohol

This isn't about cutting out everything forever; it's about giving your body a reset, not a sentence.

When gut and liver function improve, some foods may be reintroduced with no issues. The key is lowering the **total inflammatory load,** so your body isn't constantly reacting to what you're putting in. And when you do, your body can finally stop fighting and start thriving.

Simple, Doable Strategies to Reduce Bloat and Inflammation

You don't need a restrictive cleanse or a thirty-day gut reset to start feeling better. Most women I work with are already doing a lot, and their bodies are asking for *support*, not more stress.

Here are some of the most effective (and doable) strategies to reduce bloating, puffiness, and inflammation without flipping your life upside down.

Support Digestion

When digestion is sluggish or incomplete, bloating is inevitable, no matter how healthy you're eating. Help your body break things down so you can absorb what you're eating.

- **Digestive bitters** before meals stimulate stomach acid and bile flow.
- **Chew thoroughly** at least twenty times per mouthful. Basically, chew like your life depends on it (because your bloating kind of does).
- **Take digestive enzymes** if needed (especially with protein- or fat-heavy meals).
- **Eat without distractions** so your body stays in rest-and-digest mode.

Gentle Liver Support

Your liver is not just a detox organ; it's your inflammation filter. When it's overloaded, everything gets backed up: hormones, digestion, and toxins.

You don't need to suffer through a juice cleanse that makes you hate life. Your liver just wants some breathing room:

- **Warm lemon water in the morning** to stimulate bile flow
- **Cruciferous vegetables** (broccoli, cabbage, arugula) to support detox pathways
- **Beets and dandelion tea** to nourish and gently stimulate the liver
- **Castor oil packs** over the liver area to support lymphatic flow
- **Epsom salt baths or sweating** (sauna, walking, movement) to aid elimination

---

Want more simple, gentle ways to support your liver— without going on a restrictive detox?

Scan the QR code below or visit https://YourMidlife BodyCode.com/bonuses to download your **Liver Support Toolkit**. Inside, you'll find:

- Everyday foods that support bile flow and detox
- Easy ways to reduce toxin exposure (without perfection)
- Claudine's favorite liver-friendly meals, teas, and self-care rituals

When your liver flows, you glow!

Reduce Inflammatory Load from Food

This isn't about cutting out everything forever; it's about reducing the things that pour fuel on the fire *right now* so your body can calm down and reset.

- **Try a break from gluten and dairy**—two of the most common inflammation triggers.
- **Skip the nightly glass of wine**—Even if it's "clean," your liver still has to deal with it. Sorry, I don't make the rules!
- **Be mindful of refined sugar**—especially when stress is high or sleep is poor.
- **Focus on whole, nutrient-dense meals**—to keep your blood sugar stable.
- **Drink enough water** (with minerals)—to help flush inflammatory byproducts.

You're not weak for reacting to food; you're inflamed. And inflammation changes everything.

From Puffy & Bloated to Clear & Light

Remember Lorena, the one who was thrilled when her rings finally slipped back on? That wasn't just a cute milestone. It was her first real sign that the inflammation was starting to shift. When she came to me, she felt inflamed *everywhere*. Her face looked puffy, her stomach felt swollen after almost every meal, and her joints were achy and stiff. She kept saying, "I'm doing everything right, so why do I still feel awful in my body?"

We started slow—nothing extreme. We supported her digestion, gave her liver a little love, and pulled back on a few inflammatory foods (yes, including her girls' night cocktails). We also cleaned up a few "healthy" habits that weren't working for her.

Within weeks, the puffiness started going down. Her belly was flatter, her skin was clearer, and she wasn't constantly adjusting her clothes to feel comfortable. The number on the scale didn't change much (at first), but how she felt in her body absolutely did.

You're Not Stuck—You're Inflamed

If you've been staring in the mirror, wondering why your body feels so different lately (more bloated, more puffy, more uncomfortable), you're not imagining it. And you're not damaged. This isn't about age, laziness, or willpower. This is your body raising its hand, asking for support.

Inflammation and bloating aren't just random annoyances. They're real signs that your gut, liver, or immune system is overloaded. And the reality is, you don't need to overhaul your life to turn the dial down. Small, strategic changes, like supporting digestion, easing the burden on your liver, and lowering your inflammatory load, can help you feel clearer, lighter, and more like yourself again.

So, before you double down on dieting or cut out one more food group, take a breath. Your body isn't holding onto fat out of spite. It's holding onto *fluid* to protect you. And once that inflammation starts to go down, everything else starts to feel easier, including weight. Which brings us to our next stop.

In the next chapter, we're going to tackle one of the most frustrating midlife mysteries of all: the weight that won't budge. You'll learn why it's not about eating less or working out more. It's about restoring balance where your body needs it most. Let's decode that next.

TL;DR — Chapter 7: The Puffy, Bloated, Inflamed Puzzle

- Puffiness isn't just "weight gain." It's often bloating and inflammation, two different but connected issues.
- Bloating comes from sluggish digestion and trapped gas, often driven by gut imbalances, food sensitivities, or low stomach acid.
- Inflammation is systemic, showing up as puffiness, swelling, or water retention when the immune system is on overload.
- Gut dysfunction, liver congestion, and hidden food triggers are the most common drivers.
- Reducing your inflammatory load (not chasing perfection) helps your body calm down and release the excess fluid.
- Simple, sustainable shifts like digestive support, gentle liver care, and mindful food choices make a noticeable difference.

Bottom line: You're not stuck, you're inflamed. When your body feels safe and supported, it lets go of the puff, the water, and the weight.

Chapter 8: The Stubborn Weight Story

The weight won't budge, but that doesn't mean you've failed.

If eating less and exercising more were the answers, you wouldn't be reading this chapter. You've already done all that. You've cut carbs, counted calories, flirted with fasting, and pushed yourself through workouts when you were already running on fumes. And yet ... the scale won't budge. Or worse, it creeps up no matter what you do.

It's infuriating. Disheartening. And maybe even a little scary. But here's the reframe I want to offer you: It's not that your body is failing; it's that your body is trying to *protect* you.

Yes, really.

We've been conditioned to treat stubborn weight like a personal flaw. Like it's a sign that you're doing something wrong or not trying hard enough. But what if that weight gain, especially around the belly, isn't about willpower or discipline at all? What if it's a symptom? What if your body isn't working *against* you but *for* you, based on the signals it's getting?

Let's start unpacking those signals (and giving you solutions), so you can finally stop blaming yourself and start making real, sustainable progress.

Midlife Weight Is a Symptom, Not a Personal Failing

The truth is weight gain in midlife isn't just about calories in versus calories out. Your metabolism is far more complex than a math equation. Fat storage, particularly around the belly, is often a biological survival response. Your body holds onto weight when it senses:

- Blood sugar instability
- Chronic stress or emotional overwhelm
- Shifting hormone levels
- Inflammation or toxic burden

This isn't dysfunction. It's *adaptation*. If your body feels under threat—nutritionally, emotionally, environmentally—it's going to do what it's designed to do: conserve energy, store fuel, and prioritize survival. That means gaining or holding onto weight isn't a mistake. It's *feedback*. And once you understand what your body is reacting to, you can shift the signals it's receiving. That's the key.

Because stubborn weight isn't about a lack of willpower. It's about an overwhelmed system. And when we address what's overwhelming your system (physiologically *and* emotionally), your body can finally start to let go.

The Key Drivers of Stubborn Midlife Weight

Let's get one thing straight: Your body is not simply "holding on to fat" for no reason. It's responding intelligently and predictably to the signals it's receiving. And midlife just happens to be the perfect storm of those signals stacking up. The following are the biggest culprits driving weight gain in this season of life and what you need to know to start shifting the pattern.

Insulin Resistance: The Silent Weight Saboteur

At the center of stubborn weight (especially the kind that gathers around your belly) is often a blood sugar imbalance called insulin resistance. In plain English, this means your cells aren't responding as efficiently to insulin, the hormone that helps shuttle glucose into your cells for energy. When this happens, your body stores more fat, especially visceral fat around the organs.

But here's what most people don't realize: **You don't need to be eating sugar all day to develop insulin resistance**. Chronic stress, poor sleep, overexercising, under-eating, hormonal shifts, and even inflammation can make your body more insulin resistant, even if you're eating "clean." It's not just about food. It's about how your entire system is functioning.

And once that resistance is in play, your body has a harder time burning fat—even when you're doing everything "right." You can't outwork insulin resistance. You have to outsmart it.

Cortisol: The Belly Fat Connection

When your body perceives stress—whether it's emotional, physical, or even from excessive exercise—it pumps out cortisol, your main stress hormone. And cortisol's job is to keep you alive in a perceived emergency. That means prioritizing fast energy (glucose), storing fat for future emergencies, and putting repair, digestion, and fat-burning on the back burner.

Now imagine this happening every day. You're juggling work, caregiving, and your family's emotional load and maybe skipping meals or pushing through intense workouts in the name of "health." Your body doesn't see a fitness queen; it sees a survival situation. And when your body thinks it's in survival mode, it's going to hold onto its energy stores. This is why more effort doesn't always equal more results. In fact, sometimes it makes things worse.

Hormonal Shifts: The Hidden Weight Drivers

Estrogen and progesterone don't just influence your cycle, they impact where you store fat, how efficiently you metabolize food, and even how inflamed you are. As progesterone begins to decline in perimenopause, it creates a relative estrogen dominance, where estrogen becomes more dominant even if both hormones are technically dropping. That shift can increase fat storage (especially in the hips, thighs, and belly), slow down metabolism, and ramp up inflammation, all of which make it harder to lose weight, even with perfect habits.

Testosterone also plays a role. Even though women make far less of it than men, it helps maintain lean muscle, support metabolism, and protect libido. When testosterone declines in midlife, women may notice their muscle tone fading, weight creeping up, and desire dropping.

Your weight story is often a hormone story first. And while you can't stop your hormones from shifting, you *can* influence how your body adapts to those shifts.

When Desire Disappears

Low libido is one of the most common (yet least talked about) midlife shifts. And it is not "all in your head." Declining testosterone, changing estrogen levels, and even rising cortisol can all chip away at desire. Add in fatigue, poor sleep, and the mental load women carry, and it is no wonder intimacy can feel like one more chore.

What you can do:

- **Support testosterone naturally.** Strength training, adequate protein, and healthy fats all help maintain lean muscle and hormone balance.
- **Prioritize sleep and nervous system support.** Exhaustion and a stressed-out nervous system are two of the biggest libido killers.
- **Address vaginal dryness.** Local estriol drops or lubricants can make intimacy comfortable again.
- **Look at the big picture.** When you stabilize blood sugar, reduce hidden inflammation, and re-nourish minerals, desire often returns as your body feels safe again.

Low libido isn't permanent or "just part of getting older." It's your body's signal that it needs deeper support. When you realign your foundation, desire and connection often return naturally.

Nervous System Dysregulation: The "Wired But Tired" Loop

If you've ever felt tired but unable to relax or like your body is revving at a hundred miles an hour while your brain is stuck in molasses, that's nervous system dysregulation in action. And it absolutely plays a role in stubborn weight. When your body is stuck in fight-or-flight mode, your metabolism slows down. It's not a glitch; it's protective. Your body assumes that now is *not* a safe time to lose its energy reserves, so it hangs on to them, even if you're in a calorie deficit.

This is why calming your nervous system isn't just a "nice to have." It's a *requirement* for weight release. Your body won't shed weight if it doesn't feel safe. Full stop.

Why Overexercising & Undereating Backfire

If you've ever responded to weight gain by tightening the reins—cutting calories even more, skipping meals, or doubling down on workouts—you're not alone. That's the strategy we've been taught since forever: eat less, move more, and the weight will come off. But here's the hard truth most women in midlife eventually realize (usually through painful trial and error): the harder you push, the harder your body resists.

Extreme dieting and excessive exercise don't reset your metabolism; they stress it out. And that stress isn't just emotional, it's physiological. When you undereat or overtrain, especially without proper recovery, you trigger a survival response in the body. Cortisol levels rise, blood sugar becomes harder to regulate, and your body starts conserving energy instead of burning it.

It doesn't matter that you're eating "healthy" or crushing it at the gym. If your nervous system is fried and your tank is bone dry, your body sees these as threats, and it responds the way it's wired to—by slowing your metabolism, stashing fat for later, and putting weight loss dead last on the priority list.

The solution isn't deprivation, it's nourishment. That doesn't mean throwing discipline out the window. It means supporting your body, so it feels safe enough to let go. Instead of punishing your body into submission, you coax it back into balance with enough food, enough rest, and the right kind of movement at the right time.

You can't bully your body into balance. And you don't need to. You just need to shift the inputs, so your body no longer thinks it needs to protect you by holding on to every ounce.

Practical Strategies for Sustainable Weight Release

The section you've been waiting for!

If your body has been holding on to excess weight, it's not because you're not trying hard enough; it's because it hasn't felt safe enough to let go. That means the most effective approach isn't about restriction or punishment; it's about regulation, nourishment, and support. Let's shift from trying to force weight off to giving your body what it needs to release it.

Balance Your Blood Sugar

Keeping blood sugar stable is one of the fastest ways to calm the body's emergency signals and reduce fat storage. Some of these have been alluded to in previous chapters, but here's the full list to stabilize blood sugar so your body can feel steady, rather than stressed:

- **Aim for twenty to thirty grams of protein per meal**. Protein is your blood sugar stabilizer, muscle preserver, and appetite regulator. It sets the tone for how the rest of your meal is processed.
- **Eat within an hour of waking**. No more skipping breakfast or "running on coffee." Your body needs fuel early to feel safe.
- **Stick to consistent meal timing.** Going too long between meals can spike cortisol and make insulin resistance worse. Regular meals = steady fuel.
- **Ditch the excessive fasting.** Intermittent fasting can work for some people, but for many midlife women, fasting too long sends the body into stress mode. A twelve- to fourteen-hour overnight fast is usually plenty.

Want help putting this into action?

I created the **Bye-Bye Stubborn Weight Meal Plan** to show you what balanced blood sugar actually looks like—no guesswork required. It's packed with easy, satisfying meals that follow my anti-inflammatory, midlife-friendly guidelines (and yes, they're easy and delicious!).

Scan the QR code below or go to https://YourMidlife BodyCode.com/bye-bye to download your copy, and start fueling your body for steady energy and sustainable fat loss.

Support Your Nervous System

You don't need more willpower; you need more regulation.

- **Opt for gentler movement like walking or strength training**. These help build lean muscle and support metabolism without spiking stress hormones the way HIIT or endless cardio can.
- **Build in daily downshifts**. Breathwork, time in nature, music, laughter, silence, journaling. These aren't luxuries; they're tools for nervous system repair.
- **Create safety cues**. A warm meal, a cozy blanket, a consistent bedtime. These small signals tell your body it's OK to exhale.

Reduce Inflammation, Gently

You don't need a crash detox; you need to remove what's adding fuel to the fire.

- **Cut back on the big offenders:** gluten, dairy, refined sugar, alcohol, processed foods, seed oils. No need to go extreme, just reduce the load. Think anti-inflammatory, not anti-joy.
- **Support your gut and liver:** They're your detox team. If they're overwhelmed (from mold, pathogens, food sensitivities, toxins), it can stall progress. Be sure to download the **Liver Support Toolkit** listed in the last chapter for ideas and suggestions.
- **Prioritize rest and stress release:** Sleep and emotional decompression are both profoundly anti-inflammatory. Make space for both.

Mold: The Hidden Saboteur

While it's not the case for everyone, mold exposure is a hidden weight-loss saboteur I see more often than you'd think.

Even if you haven't had recent water damage or visible mold, past exposures (from years ago!) can linger in your system and keep your body in a chronic state of alarm. Mold toxins (called *mycotoxins*) can inflame the gut, disrupt hormones, burden the liver, trigger thyroid dysfunction, and completely throw off your nervous system's sense of safety.

In other words: **Mold can quietly sabotage all the systems that affect your weight, energy, mood, and metabolism**.

This is a deep topic—one that could fill a book on its own (and many already have). I'll include some of my favorite resources in the back of this book if this is something you want to explore further.

Optimize Sleep & Recovery

Sleep is your body's fat-burning secret weapon.

- **Aim for seven to nine hours** (and quality matters). If you're wired at night and dragging by day, that's a red flag your hormones and nervous system need support.
- **Create a wind-down routine.** Screens off, lights dim, blood sugar balanced, all set the stage for your body to truly rest.
- **Address sleep disruptors.** Blood sugar crashes, cortisol spikes, pain, and inflammation can all mess with your sleep. We'll go deeper into this in the next chapter.

If you'd give anything for a good night's sleep but can't seem to make it happen, you're in luck! That is the subject of the next chapter, so stay tuned for more tools and tips to getting your Zs.

Shift Your Mindset

This is big. You're not here to punish your body, you're here to learn how to work with it.

- **Ditch the shame and hustle mentality.** "No pain, no gain" doesn't work here. Nourishment, not deprivation, is what moves the needle.
- **Focus on consistency, not perfection.** Your body responds to safety and routine, not extremes.
- **Build trust with your body.** When you stop treating it like the enemy, it stops acting like one.

Client Case Study: When the Body Feels Safe, It Lets Go

Remember Hannah from Chapter 2? She was the woman who couldn't sleep, felt inflamed from the inside out, and was stuck in what she called "a constant state of tension." Weight loss wasn't her goal. She just wanted to stop feeling like her body was fighting her every step of the way. But as we worked on calming her nervous system, balancing her blood sugar, and supporting her body instead of pushing it ...

Eighteen pounds came off—*without* changing her diet.

No tracking. No overhauling her meals. No intense workouts. Just a shift in how her body *felt* and how it finally felt *safe* to let go. Because when your nervous system isn't in overdrive, your body stops clinging to weight for dear life. That's the shift most women miss when they're stuck in "try harder" mode. And for Hannah, it changed everything.

You're Not Failing—Your Body Is Communicating

Your weight is not your worth. It's a signal. And when you stop blaming your body and start listening to what it's trying to tell you, everything changes. That stubborn weight isn't a sign that you're doing something wrong; it's a sign that your body's overwhelmed, undersupported, or on high alert.

And here's the amazing thing: You have the power to shift the signals.

When you stop punishing and start nourishing ...

When you stop overworking and start restoring ...

When you create safety instead of stress ...

Your body can finally exhale. And that's when it lets go ... of weight, inflammation, exhaustion, and all the old stories that told you your worth was tied to your size.

You don't need to be fixed.

You just need better inputs.

And one of the most overlooked (but *hugely* important) inputs your body responds to is sleep. If you've ever stared at the ceiling at eleven p.m. or three a.m., wired *and* exhausted, wondering why your brain won't shut off ... the next chapter is for you.

TL;DR: Chapter 8—The Stubborn Weight Story

- Midlife weight gain isn't failure; it's your body's survival response to blood sugar swings, stress, hormone shifts, and inflammation.
- Insulin resistance is a key driver. You can't out-diet or out-exercise it—you have to stabilize blood sugar and lower hidden stressors.
- Cortisol and nervous system overload drive belly fat storage. If your body doesn't feel safe, it won't let go.
- Hormonal shifts (estrogen, progesterone, testosterone) reshape metabolism, muscle tone, and fat storage.

- Overexercising and undereating backfire, slowing metabolism and telling your body to hold on to weight.
- Practical shifts—balanced blood sugar, nervous system support, anti-inflammatory focus, quality sleep, and a mindset reset—are what unlock sustainable weight release.

Bottom line: Stubborn weight is feedback, not failure. When you stabilize blood sugar, calm your system, reduce inflammation, rest, and change the way you treat your body, it finally feels safe enough to let go.

Bonus: Don't forget to download the **Bye-Bye Stubborn Weight Meal Plan** for recipes and food strategies that support blood sugar and hormone balance.

Chapter 9: Sleep, Mood & the 3 a.m. Wake-Up Call

Newsflash: You can't out-hustle exhaustion.

If you've been feeling like your body is working against you—holding on to weight, resisting your usual routines—you're not imagining it. And chances are, the exhaustion, irritability, and restless nights are right there with it. Because when your body is under pressure, it doesn't just show up on the scale; it shows up in your sleep. In your mood. In how tightly wound you feel and how close to tears you are when someone asks what's for dinner. That's not weakness. That's biology.

The Familiar Struggle

You crawl into bed exhausted, but your brain won't turn off. Or maybe you fall asleep just fine, but like clockwork, you're wide awake at three a.m. Staring at the ceiling. Again. And when your alarm finally goes off, it feels like you're dragging yourself through molasses: foggy, groggy, and already behind before the day even begins.

The sleep struggle is frustrating enough on its own, but paired with mood swings, snapping at your partner for breathing too loudly, tearing up at a commercial, or suddenly losing your patience over the smallest thing ... it's easy to start questioning yourself.

What is wrong with me?

Why can't I just calm down?

Am I losing it?

Let me say this clearly: *Your symptoms are real, and they have a root.*

You're dealing with a **physiological imbalance**—one that is affecting your sleep, your mood, and your ability to feel like yourself. And until your body gets the support it needs, it's going to keep sounding the alarm.

The Sleep-Mood Connection & Why It's All Tied Together

It's not just that poor sleep makes you cranky or that bad moods make it harder to rest. Sleep and mood are biologically intertwined: When one starts to unravel, the other usually follows. That's because both are deeply affected by the same internal systems. If those systems are out of sync, your body won't be able to rest or regulate, no matter how many sleep hygiene tricks you try.

Here are a few of the biggest players in that internal orchestra:

- **Blood sugar stability.** Big spikes and crashes (especially at night) can wake you up, make you anxious, and leave you exhausted the next morning, even if you technically stayed in bed for eight hours.
- **Liver function.** Your liver is busiest detoxing between **one and three a.m.,** and if it's overburdened (by alcohol, medications, toxins, or hormone clearance), it can literally jolt you awake. Ever feel like your eyes fly open in the middle of the night for no reason? That could be your liver trying to catch up.
- **Hormonal shifts.** This one is huge. As progesterone declines in perimenopause, many women feel more anxious, edgy, or weepy. Add in surging cortisol and fluctuating estrogen, and you've got the perfect storm for both **sleep disturbances** and **emotional volatility**.

And here's something not enough people talk about: As estrogen declines, it doesn't just mess with your cycle; it can also affect **your airway**. Research shows that estrogen helps keep the airway flexible and, when levels drop, women can become more prone to **snoring, poor breathing, and even sleep apnea** during midlife.[13]

- **Nervous system regulation.** Your nervous system is supposed to cycle between "go mode" (fight-or-flight) and "rest-and-repair" mode. But when chronic stress, overstimulation, and burnout take over, your body gets stuck in **high alert,** making it nearly impossible to fall asleep, stay asleep, or feel calm during the day. **You might feel "tired but wired," wide awake at three a.m., or reactive to things that never used to rattle you.** That's not just emotional. It's a physiological loop driven by your brain, your body, and your environment.

On top of that, **melatonin production also drops** significantly after menopause,[14] and that is a big deal! Melatonin isn't just a supplement; it's a hormone your body naturally makes to regulate your sleep-wake cycle. Less melatonin = **less deep, restorative sleep**, especially REM and slow-wave (deep) sleep, which are crucial for emotional processing and brain repair. Even during perimenopause, shifting hormone signals and disrupted circadian rhythms can start to interfere with melatonin's natural rhythm—making quality sleep harder to come by.

So even if you *technically* sleep through the night, you may be spending more time in **light sleep**, which leaves you feeling just as tired, foggy, and irritable as if you hadn't slept at all.

---

[13] Vishal R. Tandon, Sudhaa Sharma, Annil Mahajan, et al., "Menopause and Sleep Disorders," *Journal of Mid-Life Health* 13, no. 1 (2022): 26-33, https://pubmed.ncbi.nlm.nih.gov/35707298/.
[14] Elena Toffol, Nea Kalleinen, Jari Haukka, et al., "Melatonin in Perimenopausal and Postmenopausal Women," *Menopause* 21, no. 5 (2014): 493-500, https://doi.org/10.1097/gme.0b013e3182a6c8f3.

Curious whether hormone therapy (especially bioidentical options) could help with mood or sleep? We'll unpack that more in Chapter 11, once you've got the full picture.

Understanding Sleep Stages—What You're Missing Matters

Every night, your body cycles through multiple stages of sleep, each with its own role in restoring your brain and body. Here's a quick breakdown (see also graph, below):

- **Light Sleep (Stages 1 & 2).** These make up fifty percent of sleep. This is the transition stage where your body slows down, but you're still easily awakened.
- **Deep Sleep (Slow-Wave/Stage 3).** This is where **physical repair**, immune function, and detox happen. It's the most restorative for your **body**.
- **REM Sleep.** This is where **emotional processing**, dreaming, and memory consolidation happen. REM is essential for your **brain**.

As estrogen and melatonin drop in midlife, women tend to get **less deep and REM sleep**, and **more light sleep**, which means that, even if you are technically asleep, you're not getting the kind of sleep that actually restores you.

That's why midlife sleep struggles can feel like insomnia *plus* burnout *plus* emotional whiplash.

Your Sleep Cycle:
What Happens While You Rest

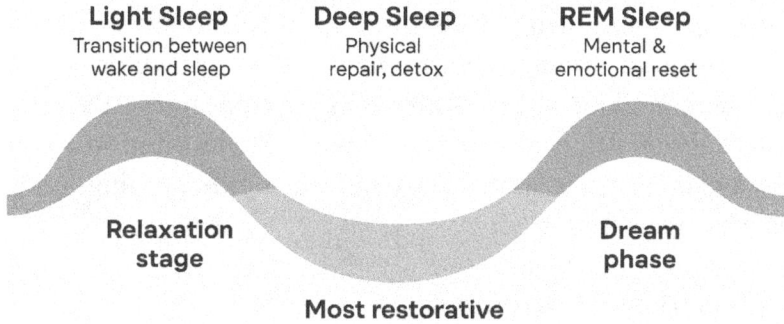

Light Sleep
Transition between
wake and sleep

Deep Sleep
Physical
repair, detox

REM Sleep
Mental &
emotional reset

Relaxation
stage

Dream
phase

Most restorative

Why the 3 a.m. Wake-Up Call Happens

So, let's talk about *that* moment. The one where your eyes snap open in the middle of the night, your mind starts racing, and no amount of deep breathing seems to help. What gives? The truth is your body isn't waking you up to torture you. It's trying to protect you. That three a.m. wake-up isn't random; it's often the result of a **chain reaction** happening behind the scenes. Here's what could be going on:

1. Blood Sugar Dips

Blood sugar instability doesn't just affect your energy or mood during the day. It can absolutely disrupt your sleep, too. When you skip meals, snack constantly, or rely on quick carbs without enough protein or fat, your blood sugar stays on a rollercoaster. By the time dinner rolls around, many women are already running on empty. If that last meal is mostly carbs, or includes wine, dessert, or something quick and unsatisfying, it often causes a sharp spike followed by a crash just a few hours later—right around the time you're trying to stay asleep. That crash might not feel dramatic during the day, but while you're sleeping, it's a different story.

When blood sugar drops too low in the middle of the night (the crash), your body sees it as a four-alarm fire. To address the "emergency" and bring levels back up, it releases your fight-or-flight hormone cortisol. The problem is that cortisol doesn't just help regulate blood sugar; it also tells your brain to wake up and be alert so you can deal with the "threat." That's often why you're wide awake at three a.m., heart racing, mind spinning, and no idea what triggered it.

2. Liver Detox Bottleneck

We've spent a lot of time talking about the liver already: how it affects your energy, your hormones, and your ability to feel like yourself. But here's where things get even more interesting: Your liver also plays a major role in your ability to sleep through the night. That's because during the overnight hours (especially between one and three a.m.), your liver kicks into its most active detox window. This is when your body is supposed to be in its deepest rest and repair mode, giving your liver space to filter out excess hormones, toxins, and metabolic waste. But if that system is overwhelmed, things start to get noisy.

Instead of quietly doing its job in the background, your liver may start sounding the alarm. And your nervous system picks up the signal. That internal "disturbance" can show up as restlessness, night sweats, vivid dreams, or a sudden wake-up with no clear reason.

This is especially common if:

- You drink alcohol in the evening
- You take medications that your body has to metabolize overnight
- You're dealing with hormone imbalances, especially during perimenopause or menopause

- You're constantly under pressure or struggle to unwind
- You eat heavy or late-night meals
- You're exposed to toxins at work, in your home, or through personal care products

You don't need to check every box for your liver to be overwhelmed. Even a few of these can create enough internal stress to trigger that three a.m. wake-up. The more overloaded your system is, the more likely your body will "tap you on the shoulder" in the middle of the night to deal with what hasn't been cleared. But once you understand this connection, you can support your body in smarter, gentler ways and *finally* get the uninterrupted sleep your system has been craving.

3. Gut Bugs Party at Night

We've already touched on how gut imbalances can impact energy, mood, and inflammation. But here's something most women don't realize: The state of your gut can also play a major role in whether you sleep through the night.

When your digestive system slows down for the night, certain bacteria, yeast, or parasites can become more active. If the gut is inflamed or out of balance, that activity can trigger internal stress signals that your body interprets as a threat. You may not feel anything in your belly, but your nervous system definitely picks up on the chaos.

This disruption can lead to:

- A spike in histamine, which stimulates alertness
- Inflammation that puts extra pressure on the liver's detox load
- Interference with calming brain chemicals like serotonin and GABA
- Signals to your body that raise your heart rate, body temp, or make you feel like you need to pee (again)

You might not connect these things to your gut at all. But if you're consistently waking up between two and four a.m., feeling hot, restless, anxious, or needing to pee multiple times—even when you didn't drink much before bed—your gut could be playing a hidden role.

Gut bugs don't always cause obvious digestive symptoms. Sometimes, they quietly irritate your system, stir up inflammation, and keep your body in a state of low-grade alert that makes deep rest nearly impossible.

Could Your Gut Be Keeping You Up?
Common Gut Clues You Might Miss

- Waking up between two and four a.m. for no clear reason
- Restless sleep or vivid, unsettling dreams
- Needing to pee multiple times overnight
- Feeling hot, itchy, or unsettled at night
- Skin flare-ups (rashes, hives, breakouts)
- Increased anxiety or irritability without a known trigger
- Sugar or carb cravings in the afternoon or evening
- Evening bloating or a waistband that suddenly feels tight
- Food sensitivities that seem to come and go
- Trouble falling or staying asleep—even with good sleep hygiene

---

4. Nervous System Hypervigilance

Your body knows how to sleep. But when your nervous system is stuck in overdrive, it's like someone's left the lights on in your internal control tower.

Even after a long, exhausting day, you may still feel wired. You're tired, but your mind is racing, your body's buzzing, or you're suddenly aware of every sound, breath, or flicker of light in the room. That's not you being dramatic. That's a **dysregulated nervous system** that hasn't been given permission to power down.

When your body spends all day in "go mode," it can forget how to switch into rest-and-repair mode. And once you're asleep, your nervous system doesn't just shut off. If it's still on high alert, it keeps scanning for threats, interruptions, or discomfort, especially during the lighter phases of sleep. That hyperawareness makes it harder to enter the **deep, restorative stages** you need to feel rested.

Even small things can trigger wake-ups in this state:

- A slight drop in blood sugar
- A liver detox signal
- A message from your gut
- A sound, temperature shift, or light leak
- A dream that gets "interpreted" as a stressor

Instead of sleeping through it, your brain says, *Nope, let's stay alert just in case.*

This can also happen when your **cortisol rhythm is out of sync,** spiking at night instead of tapering off the way it should. That inverted rhythm can elevate heart rate, body temperature, and mental chatter, making it feel like your body is fighting rest, even when you want it badly.

It's not that you're doing something wrong. It's that your body doesn't feel safe enough to fully let go. But guess what? This pattern can be changed. And no, it doesn't require perfection, willpower, or an hour of meditation every day. We'll walk through exactly how to start shifting things in the Practical Strategies section coming up. But first, let's look at how all this nighttime chaos affects your days. Because, if you've been feeling more irritable, anxious, or reactive lately, that's not random either.

Mood Swings & Irritability: The Daytime Side of the Same Coin

If your nights are restless, your days are probably reactive.

The same imbalances that are waking you up at three a.m. are the ones leaving you snappy, teary, or overwhelmed by three p.m. Mood swings, irritability, brain fog, and that "walking on eggshells" feeling aren't just emotional; they're your body's way of telling you it's still out of sync. Your mood isn't separate from your sleep. It's the next chapter in the same story.

Here's what might be driving it:

- **Blood sugar crashes.** When your blood sugar dips too low, your body releases cortisol to bring it back up. This can cause a sudden mood shift—irritability, anxiety, or even tears for no clear reason. And if it happened overnight, too? You're already starting the day on edge.

- **Mineral depletion.** Stress and disrupted sleep drain key minerals like **magnesium** and **potassium**, which help regulate your mood, focus, and nervous system function. Without them, even small stressors feel bigger than they are.

- **Hormonal shifts.** Declining **progesterone** can make you more anxious or emotionally sensitive, while **high cortisol** from poor sleep or chronic stress can make you feel on edge, wired, or angry, often without knowing why.

- **Poor sleep.** This one's obvious but powerful. Lack of deep, quality sleep affects everything—impulse control, emotional regulation, and your ability to think clearly. It also increases sugar cravings and lowers your tolerance for frustration, which is a dangerous combo when your calendar is already full.

Your mood isn't a flaw. It's feedback. Some women chalk up their irritability or brain fog to hormones. Others start to wonder if they have attention deficit hyperactivity disorder (ADHD)—especially if focus, organization, or emotional regulation feel harder than they used to. And while the rise in midlife ADHD diagnoses is very real, there's something else worth considering ...

Is it really ADHD ... or is your brain running on empty?

We've seen a huge increase in women being diagnosed with ADHD in their forties and fifties. But here's the truth: What looks like ADHD is often the result of deep physiological depletion. If your brain isn't getting the fuel, minerals, or sleep it needs, you'll naturally struggle to focus, follow through, and keep your emotions in check. That doesn't mean the label is wrong. But it *does* mean it's not the whole story.

Common ADHD-like symptoms that often have functional root causes:

- Forgetfulness or trouble following through on tasks
- Difficulty focusing or prioritizing
- Emotional outbursts or low frustration tolerance
- Restlessness or mental fatigue
- Overwhelm that leads to avoidance or shutdown

All of these can be triggered (or made worse) by things like:

- Blood sugar instability
- Poor sleep quality
- Mineral and neurotransmitter imbalances
- Hormonal shifts

- Chronic stress or nervous system dysregulation

The great news is that these patterns can shift. When your body is better supported, your brain starts working like it's supposed to. And you may find that what felt like a lifelong diagnosis was actually your body waving a flag for help.

Practical Strategies to Support Sleep & Mood

Now that we've covered what's really behind your restless nights and reactive days, let's talk about what actually helps. These aren't hacks or quick fixes. They're small, powerful shifts that help your body get back into rhythm, supporting the systems that are screaming for relief.

You don't need to do all of these at once. Choose what feels doable and start building your own nighttime rhythm. To make this easier, I created a few simple tools to help you get started.

Want to build a personalized nighttime rhythm?

Download the **Sleep & Sanity Support Kit** (https://YourMidlifeBodyCode.com/bonuses) or use QR code, below). It includes calming ideas, customizable routines, and a fill-in-the-blank nightly plan to help your body feel safe enough to rest.

Support Blood Sugar Stability

- Your sleep depends on it. If your blood sugar is swinging high and low all day or crashing in the middle of the night, your nervous system stays stuck in high alert. Don't skip meals, especially dinner. Make sure each one includes protein and healthy fats.
- Watch the "sneaky sugars" in your meals and snacks.
- Eat breakfast within sixty minutes of waking, even if it's light.
- Avoid eating two to three hours before bedtime, unless you tend to wake up around three a.m.
- If you do wake up at that time, try a small bedtime snack with protein and fat (like a spoonful of almond butter or a hard-boiled egg with sea salt). It can help anchor your blood sugar through the night.

Lighten the Liver's Load

Your liver's detox window is between one and three a.m. If it's overwhelmed, you'll feel it, often with restlessness, wake-ups, or night sweats.

- Sip dandelion tea or warm lemon water in the afternoon
- Load your plate with cruciferous veggies like broccoli, cabbage, or arugula
- Avoid alcohol close to bedtime
- Try castor oil packs a few times a week to support gentle detox pathways
- Take a detox bath or foot soak one to two hours before bed to raise body temp, then cool down—mimicking your body's natural sleepy-time rhythm

- Consider magnesium before bed to support both detox and nervous system regulation

Downshift Your Nervous System

Your body can't slam on the brakes at bedtime if it's been in go-mode all day. Nervous system downshifting needs to happen in **small doses throughout the day**, not just at night.

- Build in a calming evening routine with low lights and no screens
- Try breathwork, stretching, or journaling as a pre-bed signal
- Use calming "mini resets" during the day: step outside, shake it out, stretch, or do a few rounds of box breathing
- Reference the **Sleep & Sanity Support Kit** for calming tools and gentle nervous system support you can use day or night

Gentle Hormone Support

You don't need to jump straight to hormone replacement to start seeing shifts. Small changes can help your body recalibrate.

- Prioritize gut health with hormone-friendly foods (fiber, healthy fats, cruciferous veggies)
- Try seed cycling (rotating specific seeds like flax, pumpkin, sunflower, and sesame to gently support estrogen and progesterone balance) or gentle adaptogens like ashwagandha or rhodiola if appropriate
- Work with a practitioner to explore natural progesterone or other sleep support (herbal or bioidentical), if needed

- Be cautious with melatonin supplements, sleeping pills, or even CBD. They can be helpful, but they're often a band-aid when your body is missing deeper support.

Build Daily Sleep-Boosting Rituals

Getting good sleep starts long before bedtime. The things you do *all day long* are what help your body feel safe enough to fully rest at night.

Here are simple habits that prime your brain and body for deeper sleep:

- **Get sunlight early.** Go outside within thirty to sixty minutes of waking. Even cloudy-day light helps regulate your circadian rhythm.
- **Move daily.** Walk, stretch, dance, whatever works for you. Movement signals safety to the nervous system and balances energy.
- **Stay consistent.** Wake up and go to bed around the same time each day, even on weekends, to support your body's natural clock.
- **Start winding down early.** About sixty to ninety minutes before bed, begin turning off screens, dimming lights, and shifting into calm.
- **Use rituals that feel good.** Stretching, journaling, light reading, gratitude lists, or calming tea all tell your body it's safe.
- **Make your bedroom a sanctuary.**
    - Cool the room (aim for 64–67°F). Use a cooling bed pad (I recommend Chilipad®) or Chillow pillow, if needed.
    - Use blackout curtains
    - Declutter your space
    - Try a lavender diffuser or calming essential oils

- **Explore other tools.** Try foot massage, binaural beats, cognitive behavioral therapy (CBT) for insomnia, or acupressure.
- **Use sound as support.** Listen to calming audiobooks, white noise, or "nothing happens" stories to help you drift off.

If you're still struggling, it might be time to work with a functional practitioner to look at root causes like gut health, hormones, or toxins.

Get the checklist and more details in the **Sleep & Sanity Support Kit** (grab it at https://YourMidlifeBodyCode.com/bonuses).

This isn't about doing all the right things perfectly. It's about giving your body the signals, support, and consistency it's been craving. Every step you take toward regulation, during the day and at night, gives your body a chance to feel safe enough to rest, recover, and rebalance.

A Word of Caution on Sleep Aids

It's tempting to reach for melatonin, sleeping pills, or even CBD to "fix" your sleep, but they often act as a band-aid instead of addressing the deeper reasons your body isn't sleeping well.

Here's what you might not know:

Melatonin
- Many sleep issues are not due to melatonin deficiency. Adding more may not be the answer.
- Supplements aren't strictly regulated—dosages vary widely, and what's on the label may not be accurate.
- Long-term use can blunt your body's own melatonin production.

- Most melatonin is produced in the **gut**, so supporting digestion and gut health is essential.

Sleeping Pills
- Many come with serious side effects, including **rebound insomnia** (worse sleep when you stop).
- Can often cause dependency, physical or psychological.
- If you're taking them, work with a provider before stopping. Use lifestyle, nutrition, and natural tools alongside as you taper.

CBD
- May help you fall asleep, but over time, it can interfere with deep, restorative sleep and lead to more nighttime wake-ups.
- Chronic use has also been linked to liver and thyroid stress in some studies.

The real fix starts with supporting your nervous system, gut, and hormones, not suppressing symptoms.

From 3 a.m. Zombie to Rested & Resilient

At fifty-five years old, Natalie had tried everything to fix her sleep: bioidentical hormones, antidepressants, therapy, and a rotating list of supplements. But she still couldn't fall asleep without a nightly dose of three CBD/THC gummies. Even then, she often woke at three a.m. with her heart pounding. Her moods were unpredictable, her digestion was a mess, and she felt stuck in a cycle she couldn't escape.

A few strategic but powerful shifts were *finally* able to help her move the needle. We added a bedtime protein-fat snack to balance her blood sugar, introduced a gentle digestive enzyme to take the pressure off her gut, and built in five-minute nervous system "reset" breaks during the day—before her body hit overload. These simple tweaks gave her body the safety it needed to downshift at night. Within weeks, she was sleeping deeper, waking less, and feeling emotionally steadier. Her energy came back, her digestion smoothed out, and, best of all, she felt like *herself* again instead of a passenger in her own life.

You don't have to accept restless nights, emotional rollercoasters, or that "wired but tired" feeling as your new normal. Your body isn't broken; it's just been overloaded. The fantastic bit is that you now have the tools to start listening, supporting, and shifting.

And we're just getting started!

In the next section, we'll move from decoding your symptoms to reprogramming your body for real, sustainable results. This is where it all starts to come together, and you start to feel like *you* again.

TL;DR: Chapter 9—Sleep, Mood, & the 3 a.m. Wake-Up Call

- Midlife sleep and mood struggles aren't random; they stem from the same imbalances.
- Blood sugar dips, liver overload, hormonal shifts, gut bugs, and a nervous system stuck in "go mode" all drive the three a.m. wake-up.
- Poor sleep feeds mood swings, irritability, and brain fog, and emotional strain makes deep sleep harder—a cycle you *can* break.
- Melatonin, sleeping pills, or CBD don't address the root causes and can even backfire long-term.

- Gentle support during the day (steady meals, liver care, nervous system resets) sets you up for deeper, restorative sleep at night.
- Simple rituals (consistent bedtime, wind-down routines, movement, mineral and protein support) make the biggest difference.

Bottom line: You're not broken or weak; your body is overloaded. Once you support the roots, sleep and mood begin to stabilize.

Part 3: Reclaim

You've made it through the noise, the doubt, the "What's wrong with me?" spiral. You've decoded the symptoms, realigned the systems, and started giving your body the support it's been craving. Now, it's time to reclaim your energy, your clarity, your **resilience**, *and* your **trust in yourself**.

This section is about forward momentum. Not by doing more or pushing harder but by making smarter, simpler choices that work for *you*. You'll learn how to stop chasing health trends and start making confident, targeted shifts based on what your body needs most right now.

You don't need to be perfect. You don't need to do everything. You just need a path that makes sense and the clarity to follow it. With the right tools and a plan that fits your real life, you can feel better in your body than you have in years.

You've already done the hardest part. Now it's time to move forward with confidence.

Chapter 10: Personalized Tweaks, Not Overhauls

Sometimes, all it takes is a pinch of salt.

You've already done so much heavy lifting. You've decoded your symptoms, started to regulate your systems, and learned how to *listen* to your body instead of second-guessing it. Now we shift into something even more powerful: refinement. This is where things start to feel lighter—not because you're doing more but because you're doing what actually matters.

You don't need a seventy-five-step protocol or a total overhaul. In fact, trying to do everything is often what keeps you stuck. Sometimes, all it takes is the right tweak in the right place, like a pinch of salt that brings the whole meal into balance. That's the power of personalization. And it's what this chapter is all about.

We're going to help you figure out what your body needs *most* right now. Then make small, strategic shifts that support exactly that—the few shifts your body *actually needs* right now. That's what creates momentum. Because this phase isn't about chasing perfection. It's about building something sustainable and *powerful*.

The Power of Small, Strategic Tweaks

"Great acts are made up of small deeds."[15] *- Lao Tzu*

It's easy to assume that big results require big changes. That if you're not overhauling your meals, logging ten thousand steps,

---

[15] Lao Tzu, *Tao Te Ching*, Translated by Stephen Mitchell, (Harper Perennial Modern Classics, 2006).

or taking a whole shelf of supplements, you're not doing "enough." But the most powerful shifts often come from the **smallest, most targeted changes**, especially when they're based on what your body needs.

Think of this as your "bring-it-into-balance" phase. These aren't random hacks or trendy protocols. They're strategic adjustments rooted in your body's signals, designed to relieve what's overloading you, replenish what's missing, and rebalance what's off track.

When you support your body's actual priorities:

- Symptoms start to settle
- Energy stabilizes
- Mood lifts
- Sleep deepens
- That sense of internal chaos starts to quiet

And it doesn't take doing everything at once. One woman might need nervous system support first. Another might need liver support. Someone else might just need more minerals and blood sugar consistency to feel dramatically better.

It's the difference between doing more and doing what actually works. Because sometimes, just the right shift—like a pinch of salt—can bring everything into harmony.

How to Identify Your Priorities (without Guessing)

If you've ever felt overwhelmed by your symptoms—unsure where to start, what to fix first, or whether it even *matters*—you're not alone. But here's the exciting part: Your body is already telling you what it needs. You just need to know how to listen.

Start by looking at your top one or two most dominant symptoms—not the full list, just the ones shouting loudest right now. That's your entry point. Addressing the clearest signals often creates ripple effects you can feel across your entire system.

Here's what that might look like:

- **Chronic fatigue?** Start with minerals and blood sugar regulation. These are foundational for energy and stress resilience.
- **Bloating or puffiness?** Focus on gut and liver support first. That can calm inflammation and improve detox.
- **Mood swings and three a.m. wake-ups?** Begin with nervous system regulation and blood sugar stability. These shifts help restore safety and rhythm.

You don't need to fix everything at once. You just need to **focus on the loudest signal**. Support that and watch how other things begin to fall into place.

It's like tasting a dish and knowing something's missing. You don't need to throw it out or start from scratch; you just need a pinch of the right thing to bring it into balance. That's what this step is all about. Your dominant symptoms are the signal. The right tweak is the salt.

Want help pinpointing your starting place?

Your **Symptom Decoder Guide** (https://YourMidlifeBodyCode.com/bonuses or QR code below) helps match your top symptoms to the system that needs support, so you can take action with *clarity,* not confusion.

The Art of Layering: Less is More

This is where most people get overwhelmed, thinking they need to do everything at once. But real change doesn't come from overhauls. It comes from smart layering. Just like you wouldn't dump every spice into a dish at once, you don't need to throw every health strategy at your body all at once, either. It's not about doing more, it's about knowing *what* to add, and *when*.

Start with your foundation: minerals, blood sugar, and digestion. These three set the stage for everything else. Once that's in place, you can layer in more targeted support for hormones, liver, or nervous system balance, depending on what your body is asking for most.

Respect your body's pace. Healing isn't a thirty-day sprint. Think of this as building flavor in a slow-cooked meal. Let each ingredient (or tweak) have a chance to work before adding more.

The Layering Approach: Build, Don't Overhaul

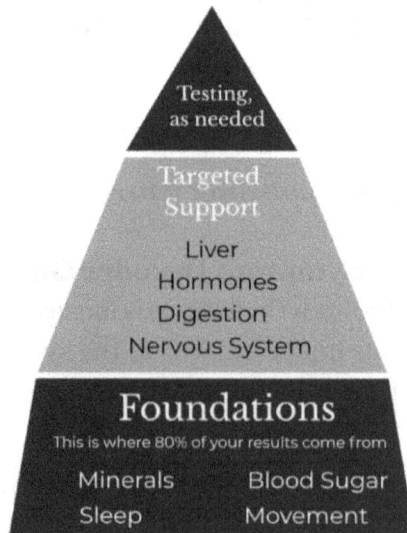

Testing, as needed

Targeted Support

Liver
Hormones
Digestion
Nervous System

Foundations
This is where 80% of your results come from

Minerals   Blood Sugar
Sleep   Movement

Build your plan from the bottom up. Start with the basics and layer only what you need, when you need it.

"Little by little, a little becomes a lot."[16] *- Tanzanian proverb*

Simple, High-Impact Tweaks You Can Actually Do

I will admit, most of the needle-movers aren't flashy. They're foundational. You've already seen how the right "pinch of salt" can bring things into balance. These are the practical ways to do that in your daily life.

You don't need to overhaul your life. Pick one or two that feel doable. Let your wins build from there.

Some of the most powerful (and underused) tweaks include:

- **Daily mineral support:** adrenal cocktails, magnesium lotion, or Epsom salt baths
- **Protein at every meal:** aim for twenty to thirty grams to anchor blood sugar and energy
- **Balanced meals:** include fat *and* fiber to avoid blood sugar swings
- **Gentle liver love:** lemon water, cruciferous veggies, castor oil packs
- **Nervous system resets:** breathwork, nature walks, unplugged time
- **Evening wind-down rituals:** calm lights, screens off, magnesium, no alcohol

These aren't drastic. But they change how you feel—fast. Because this isn't about perfect meal plans or living "the quiet life." It's about making progress while you're answering forty-seven texts, folding laundry, and figuring out who needs to be picked up where.

---

[16] Tanzanian proverb, commonly cited in collections of African proverbs, exact origin unknown.

"It's difficult to change overnight but if you are persistent and take one step at a time you will see results!"[17] *- Jack LaLanne*

Feeling ready for structure—but not more complexity?

Download the **30-Day Body Code Reset Plan** https://YourMidlifeBodyCode.com/bonuses or QR code, below) for weekly focus areas and simple daily steps. No guesswork, just momentum.

Real Life: When Small Tweaks Change Everything

You met Natalie in the last chapter: She was waking up at three a.m., burned out, and overwhelmed by everything she'd tried (and everything that hadn't worked). But those first few simple tweaks gave her something she hadn't felt in a long time: traction.

Her sleep began to stabilize. Her mood felt steadier. But the *biggest* shift was that she no longer felt like she had to fix everything all at once. Instead of jumping from supplement to supplement or spiraling in *What now?* mode, she **focused on what her body was asking for**. And it worked.

Her energy lifted, her gut calmed, and her confidence grew with every small win. For the first time in years, she felt a sense

---

[17] Jack LaLanne, *Revitalize Your Life After Fifty*, (ed. Hastings House Pub, 1995), https://libquotes.com/jack-lalanne/quote/lbe3h8s.

of *peace*. Natalie didn't have some big breakthrough moment. What changed was her focus. Once she stopped trying to do *everything* and started doing the *right* things, it all felt more doable. She wasn't drowning in options anymore. She had direction. And that changed everything.

That's the power of strategic support. When it's aligned with what your body actually needs, it's not just easier, it's more effective.

When You Want Even More Clarity

By now, you've made real progress. You've stopped trying to fix *everything* and started focusing on what actually moves the needle. And your body has responded. The truth is, a lot of women start feeling better just from these micro-adjustments, alone. You don't need fancy labs or a full protocol to make big changes. You just need the *right support in the right places*. And you've already started doing that.

But what if you've made the changes ... and some things *still* feel stuck? What if the symptoms are still tangled, or you've hit a plateau and don't know what else to try? That's where functional testing can help.

You've already learned how to listen to your body. You've made smart, strategic shifts based on what it's asking for and, in many cases, that's enough to create real change. But if your symptoms persist despite the foundational work, that doesn't mean you've failed. It means there's more data to be uncovered. Functional testing doesn't replace your instincts; it fills in the gaps. It shows you what you *can't* see on your own: hormone levels, stress patterns, detox bottlenecks, gut pathogens, and more. It takes the guesswork out of the process so you can stop spinning your wheels and start working with real clarity.

Because when you know what's really going on, you can stop chasing symptoms and *finally* address what's driving them. It's not about being "perfect" or doing more. It's about working *smarter*, not harder.

In the next chapter, I'll show you the functional tests I use most often (and why), what they reveal, and how they can help you create even more targeted support—*if* and *when* you're ready.

TL;DR: Chapter 10—Personalized Tweaks, Not Overhauls

- You don't need a complete overhaul to feel better, just small, targeted tweaks that meet your body where it is.
- The most effective shifts relieve overload, replenish what's missing, and rebalance what's off track.
- Start with your loudest symptoms. They point to your clearest priorities.
- Build layer by layer: foundations first (minerals, blood sugar, digestion), then add targeted support.
- Simple daily actions—like protein at breakfast, mineral support, gentle liver care, or nervous system resets—create powerful ripple effects.
- If symptoms persist despite these tweaks, functional testing provides the missing data.

Bottom line: Big change doesn't come from doing everything. It comes from doing what actually matters for *your* body.

Chapter 11: Lab Work That Matters (and How to Interpret It)

When lifestyle shifts haven't cracked the code, functional labs help you find the missing pieces.

Reality Check

Let's be honest: By the time most women find their way to me, they've already had their bloodwork done—more than once. Maybe your doctor ran a "full panel," and maybe you've even seen a specialist. And yet ... you're still tired. Still inflamed. Still gaining weight for no reason. Still being told everything looks "normal."

Maybe you've heard some version of this:

- "It's just stress."
- "It's your age."
- "Your labs are fine. You're just getting older."

But *you* know better. You know your body isn't just being dramatic. You can feel that something's off, but you just haven't been given the right tools to figure out what.

Here's the "aha": You're not getting the wrong answers; you're asking the wrong questions.

Why Conventional Labs Miss the Mark

Traditional lab work isn't designed to optimize your health. It's designed to catch disease once it's already there. And that leaves a *huge* gap between *technically fine* and *functionally thriving*. The ranges used on most blood panels are based on averages of the general population ... which, let's be real, isn't exactly the picture of vibrant health.

These tests can absolutely be helpful, but only when you know how to interpret them through the right lens. That's where **functional labs** come in. They're not about diagnosing disease; they're about spotting patterns of dysfunction early, before they escalate into something more serious. Functional testing helps you uncover the "why" behind your symptoms, make sense of confusing patterns, and stop wasting time on generic advice that doesn't move the needle.

In this chapter, I'll walk you through the three core functional tests I use most often in my practice, what they show, who they help, and how to use the data without getting overwhelmed. You don't need to be a practitioner to understand your body. You just need a translator who can make the data make sense.

The Problem with Conventional Labs

You can have "normal" labs on paper and still feel awful, because those ranges are designed to flag disease, not catch early dysfunction. They're based on averages from people who may already be exhausted, inflamed, or dealing with chronic conditions. That's why being "in range" doesn't mean you're in balance; it just means you haven't tripped an alarm yet. Functional labs flip the question from "Are you sick?" to "Where are things starting to break down, and why?"

Normal is not the same as optimal.

These labs also tend to look at individual markers in isolation, without connecting the dots. Let me give you an example: You might have "normal" thyroid labs (i.e., your TSH is in range), but you're still dragging through the day, your hair is falling out, your weight is creeping up, and your hands and feet are ice blocks. If no one checked your thyroid antibodies, iron levels, or mineral status, they missed the bigger picture.

Or maybe your fasting glucose looks fine, but your insulin is sky-high and you're crashing by three p.m. Again, technically normal, but functionally struggling. It's like only checking your gas gauge when your check engine light is flashing.

Conventional labs ask: *Are you sick?*

Functional labs ask: *Where are things starting to break down and why?*

That question changes everything.

What Functional Labs Actually Do

Functional lab tests aren't here to slap you with a diagnosis. They're here to show you what's going on *before* things spiral that far. Instead of asking, "Are you sick enough, yet?" these tests ask, "Where is your body struggling to keep up?" so you can address brewing issues before they become full-blown dysfunction.

They work by zooming out and identifying patterns of imbalance: how your hormones are interacting with detox pathways, how your gut health is influencing your brain and immune function, and how mineral status is affecting your energy, sleep, and blood sugar. They reveal where communication is breaking down, where stress is hitting hardest, and why your symptoms keep flaring despite your best efforts. They don't hand you a diagnosis. They hand you a roadmap.

When you can see what your body needs most right now, you can stop throwing spaghetti at the wall and start making targeted changes that move the needle. You can connect symptoms to root causes and finally shift from frustration to forward motion.

The Three Core Tests: A Full-System Overview

There are dozens of functional labs out there, but these three form the foundation. They give the clearest, most actionable view of how your body is functioning beneath the surface. If you want to stop guessing and start targeting what's actually going on, this is where you begin.

Yes, other tests like food sensitivity panels, mold and toxin screens, neurotransmitter (neuro) panels, or DNA analysis can be layered in as needed, but these three give you a complete starting picture. And if mood, motivation, anxiety, or sleep issues are a big part of your picture, I may recommend adding the neuro panel right from the start.

➤ HTMA (Hair Tissue Mineral Analysis)

Using a small sample of hair, this test reveals your mineral levels, stress pattern, and how your nervous system is handling energy production, blood sugar, hormone regulation, and more.

It goes beyond "low" or "high."It shows how your system is adapting (or struggling) under pressure. You'll see patterns that explain fatigue, burnout, insomnia, irritability, and blood sugar swings well before they show up in standard labs.

It's your body's mineral dashboard, highlighting your body's challenges and how it's coping.

➤ DUTCH Test (Hormones, Stress, and Detox Pathways)

This dried urine test gives you a *hormonal flowchart*—not just numbers, but how your body is producing, converting, and clearing hormones like estrogen, progesterone, testosterone, melatonin, and cortisol.

You'll see how your stress response is functioning, how well your detox pathways are working, and where hormonal imbalances may be contributing to symptoms like:

- Mood swings or irritability
- Poor sleep or chronic fatigue
- Stubborn belly weight
- Hot flashes or cycle changes

It helps you stop guessing and see exactly where things are getting stuck.

What's the Difference Between Hormone Therapy and Bioidentical Hormones?

Traditional hormone replacement therapy (HRT) often uses synthetic hormones or ones derived from animal sources. Bioidentical hormone therapy (BHRT), on the other hand, uses hormones that are structurally identical to the ones your body makes. They can be compounded for your unique needs or prescribed in standardized forms. While "bioidentical" sounds more natural (and is often better tolerated), it doesn't automatically mean safer or problem-free. That's why testing still matters.

If You're Using (or Considering) BHRT, Read This First.

If you've already been prescribed BHRT or you're wondering if it might help, the DUTCH test becomes even more important. It doesn't just show your hormone levels; it reveals how your body is processing, detoxifying, and balancing those hormones behind the scenes. That's key to making sure you're getting the benefit you're after and not creating new problems.

But here's what I tell every woman I work with: BHRT is a *tool*, not a cure. If your minerals are depleted, your nervous system is in overdrive, your gut is inflamed, or your liver is sluggish, adding hormones usually doesn't solve the problem. In fact, it can sometimes make things worse. Your body needs a strong foundation first. Then—and only then—can something like BHRT be layered in strategically, if it's actually needed.

I'm not anti-hormones. I'm anti-band-aid. That's why testing first, personalizing support, and getting the *whole picture* matters so much.

➤ GI-MAP (Gut Health & Digestion)

If your gut isn't working, nothing else will. This stool test evaluates digestion, pathogens (like parasites, viruses, yeast, or *H. pylori*), immune markers, inflammation, and both good and bad bacteria. Whether you're dealing with bloating, skin issues, joint pain, low immunity, or brain fog, this test often holds the missing piece.

It's like running diagnostics on your internal ecosystem: what's thriving, what's missing, and what's causing trouble.

When Mood or Motivation Are Roadblocks

If depression, anxiety, low motivation, or poor sleep are getting in the way of your progress, I often recommend adding a neuro panel alongside the three core tests. This test looks at key brain chemicals—serotonin, dopamine, GABA, and others—that influence mood, focus, drive, and sleep quality.

When these messengers are out of balance, it can feel like you're trying to run a marathon through waist-high mud—pushing hard but getting nowhere. It's exhausting and especially frustrating if you're used to being the powerhouse who gets things done. Balancing these neurotransmitters can help clear that "mud," so your brain and body work *with* you, and every step forward feels easier.

Not Sure Where to Start?

That's exactly why I created the **Functional Testing Roadmap**. It walks you through what each test reveals, when to consider them, and how to prioritize them based on your symptoms and goals.

Download your bonus **Functional Testing Roadmap** at https://YourMidlifeBodyCode.com/bonuses or use the QR code below.

When "Normal" Isn't the Whole Story: Maya's Case

When Maya came to me in her early forties, she was frustrated and burned out. Despite working out regularly and eating clean, she was gaining weight, exhausted all day, and couldn't stay focused. And with a high-pressure job, she *needed* her brain to be "on." She had even tried one of the weight-loss injectables, but nothing made a dent. Her doctor told her everything was "normal," but she knew that wasn't the full story.

So, we dug deeper.

- Her **HTMA** showed a sluggish metabolism, high calcium shell, low potassium, and signs of hidden copper toxicity—all common in cases of chronic stress and impaired detox.

- Her **GI-MAP** flagged an overgrowth of bacteria, low digestive enzymes, and high inflammation, which were likely driving her fatigue, bloating, and immune dysfunction.
- Her **DUTCH test** revealed low testosterone, sluggish estrogen detox, and high nighttime cortisol—clear signs that her nervous system was on high alert and her hormones weren't being processed efficiently.

But it was the combination of her sluggish thyroid ratio on HTMA, systemic inflammation in her bloodwork, and classic signs of immune activation that made me dig deeper. I suspected Hashimoto's (an autoimmune thyroid disorder), even though her doctor had never tested for it. Sure enough, when we ran a **full thyroid panel**, her antibodies were through the roof—over six hundred (as opposed to the usual: under ten).

These labs didn't just give us insight; they gave Maya a plan. Once we began addressing her mineral imbalances, supporting her digestion, calming her stress response, and reducing immune triggers, her energy returned. She felt more stable. And yes, the weight finally started to shift. Plus, her antibodies began to come down because her body was no longer on high alert.

Why This Isn't About Perfection (Or Over-Testing)

Functional labs aren't about chasing perfect numbers. They're about understanding your body's priorities right now. You don't need to test everything all at once. In fact, one of the biggest mistakes I see is women getting buried in pages of results without knowing what any of it actually means. That's not what we do here.

Strategic testing allows you to work *smarter*, not harder, especially when your symptoms are layered or have been brushed off as "normal." And if testing isn't available to you right now, that's OK too. You can still take meaningful steps using the tools and insights we've already covered.

This isn't about doing everything. It's about doing the *right* things at the *right* time for *your* body.

What to Do Next: Your Functional Wellness Plan

Now that you know how to listen to your symptoms and decode your body's data (whether from symptoms, bloodwork, or functional labs), it's time to get out of survival mode and into a plan that supports your body's repair.

In the next chapter, we'll walk through how to create a Functional Wellness Plan that fits your life.

No chaos. No guesswork. No extremes. Just a clear, doable structure to help you reclaim your energy and momentum.

And if testing isn't in the cards right now, don't worry. You'll still have plenty of tools to work with, no matter where you're starting from.

Want to know what your labs are really saying?

Sometimes, the first step is just making sense of the labs you already have. That's why I offer a **Root Cause Lab Review** so you can see what's really going on underneath the surface and decide your next move with confidence.

You don't have to go all-in on advanced testing to start getting answers. Many midlife symptoms show up in bloodwork long before they're ever diagnosed. If you've had recent labs but were told everything was "normal," or you want to view them through a functional lens, this review can help.

If deeper testing like HTMA or GI-MAP would provide even more clarity, we'll talk about what that looks like and how to move forward in a way that feels aligned.

🎁 **Get $50 off your Root Cause Lab Review** as a thank-you for reading this book.

☞ Scan the QR code below or visit https://YourMidlife BodyCode.com/lab-review and use code **BODYCODE50**

TL;DR—Chapter 11: Lab Work That Matters (and How to Interpret It)

- Conventional labs look for disease, not dysfunction, so "normal" results can miss what's draining you.
- Functional labs (HTMA, DUTCH, GI-MAP) uncover hidden patterns in minerals, hormones, gut health, and stress that explain why you still feel off.

- These tests don't diagnose; they provide a roadmap to guide targeted, effective action.
- Bloodwork you already have can still hold overlooked clues when viewed through a functional lens.
- Testing isn't about perfection or more data. It's about clarity, timing, and working smarter.
- When lifestyle shifts alone don't resolve symptoms, functional labs help you stop guessing and start moving forward with precision.

Bottom line: The right data doesn't just confirm what you feel; it shows you where to focus, so you can *finally* make progress.

Chapter 12: Building Your Functional Wellness Plan

#The Real Truth

Information is everywhere. You've probably read enough articles, listened to enough podcasts, and scrolled through enough "expert tips" to fill an entire library. But here's the thing: You don't need *more* information. You need a plan that actually works for **you**.

You've already uncovered what's really going on in your body. You know why you've been feeling off, and you've gathered the kind of insights most women never get—insights that connect the dots between your symptoms and what's happening beneath the surface. Now it's time to turn that clarity into action; to stop chasing every new diet, supplement, or Instagram hack; and start building a plan that fits your body, your priorities, and your life. This isn't about a massive, all-or-nothing overhaul. It's not about starting over *one more time*. It's about working with your body, not against it.

Because here's the real truth: You deserve this. You deserve to feel good in your own skin—not just *getting by*—but fully alive. You deserve mornings when you wake up clear-headed and ready, meals that fuel you without guilt or second-guessing, and nights when your head hits the pillow and your body thanks you for it. You don't have to live in constant survival mode. You don't have to accept that this is "just midlife." You now have the tools, the knowledge, and the permission to create the kind of health that lets you show up for yourself—unapologetically.

And starting now, you're going to use them. You're ready to build your plan, one layer at a time.

The Wellness Plan Pyramid: Foundation First

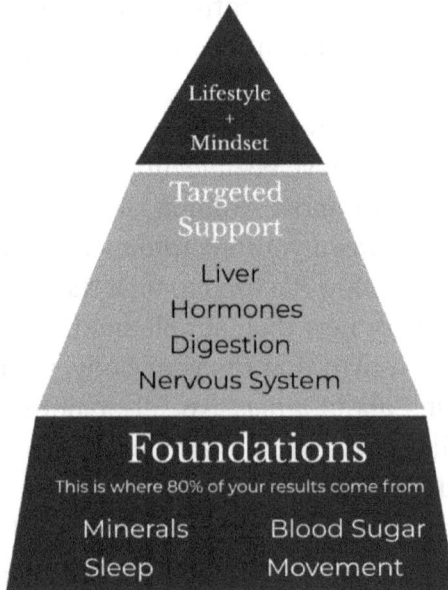

Back in Chapter 10, we talked about the Layering Approach: The idea that lasting change comes from stacking habits and supports in the right order, not from overhauling your life overnight. Now we're going to put that same concept to work in a step-by-step **Wellness Plan Pyramid**—something you can follow easily.

The Wellness Plan Pyramid: Foundation First

Lifestyle
+
Mindset

Targeted
Support

Liver
Hormones
Digestion
Nervous System

Foundations

This is where 80% of your results come from

Minerals   Blood Sugar

Sleep   Movement

Build your plan from the bottom up. No skipping steps. This is how you create lasting results.

If you're a visual learner, you may benefit from seeing this as a shape: wide at the base, narrowing as you go up. The width of each layer represents how much of your attention it should get. The Base is your day-to-day fuel and repair work. The Middle fine-tunes and addresses specific systems. The Top makes those results stick for the long haul. This pyramid isn't a "someday" plan. It's the practical framework you'll use to decide where to focus *first*, what to add *next*, and how to keep momentum without burning out.

Base Layer (Foundations)

These are your **non-negotiables**. The habits and supports that, when steady, make every other system in your body work better. If this layer is shaky, nothing built on top will last.

Non-negotiables:

- **Minerals** to spark energy, support stress resilience, and balance fluids
- **Blood sugar stability** so your energy, mood, and hormones stop yo-yoing all day
- **Sleep** that is deep and restorative so your body can repair
- **Movement** that builds strength and supports longevity without draining your reserves

When these are solid, you'll feel more grounded, more capable, and more in control. Every system above them benefits.

Middle Layer (Targeted Support)

These are the targeted, personalized supports you layer on *after* your foundations are strong.

They address specific areas like:

- **Hormones:** supporting progesterone, balancing cortisol rhythm, improving estrogen detox pathways
- **Liver:** improving detox capacity so your body processes hormones, toxins, and nutrients efficiently
- **Digestion:** optimizing stomach acid, enzyme production, and microbiome balance

- **Nervous System:** regulating your stress response so your body spends more time in "rest and repair" mode

These supports are often informed by functional testing, but even without testing, you can make progress here once your Base Layer is consistent.

Top Layer (Lifestyle + Mindset)

This is where you lock in sustainability and protect your results for the long haul.

- Set **boundaries** that protect your energy like the asset it is
- Release unnecessary stressors so your nervous system can stay regulated
- Build habits that align with your body's needs rather than external pressure or perfectionism

These shifts might not feel as urgent as "fixing symptoms," but they're what keep you from sliding back into burnout.

You build from the bottom up. No skipping steps. This is how you create results that last.

Base Layer in Action: Foundational Supports

Now, let's look at what this foundation actually includes. These aren't flashy hacks or quick fixes. They're the steady, daily supports that keep every system running smoothly. In practice, that means focusing on four essentials: minerals, blood sugar stability, restorative sleep, and movement.

Mineral Replenishment + Hydration

Minerals are like the spark plugs of your metabolism. Without them, your body can't produce energy, manage stress, or keep your nervous system steady. And most midlife women are running on empty.

- **Start simple:** add an adrenal cocktail or mineralized water in the morning
- **Soak it in:** use Epsom salt baths or foot soaks to boost magnesium
- **Eat your minerals:** prioritize mineral-rich foods like leafy greens, avocado, beets, pumpkin seeds, bone broth, and sea salt
- **Personalize if possible:** If you've done HTMA testing, use test results to target your mineral replenishment

*(See your **Mineral Support Guide** for recipes, supplement tips, and daily boosts.)*

Blood Sugar Stabilization

Balanced blood sugar is the difference between a steady, "I've got this" kind of energy and an all-day rollercoaster of crashes, cravings, and irritability. It also keeps hormones like cortisol, insulin, and estrogen from swinging wildly.

- Aim for **twenty to thirty grams of protein** at each meal
- Include healthy fat and fiber to slow the breakdown of carbs
- Avoid long gaps between meals (Most women do best eating every three to four hours.)
- Reduce inflammatory foods that spike blood sugar or disrupt gut function (Gluten, dairy, refined sugar, and alcohol are the big ones for many women.)

*(See Week 2 of your **30-Day Body Code Reset Plan** for a step-by-step guide.)*

Sleep Optimization

If you're not sleeping well, you're not recovering. Period. Sleep is when your brain processes the day, your hormones reset, and your cells repair.

- Keep a consistent bedtime and wake time (yes, even on weekends)
- Power down screens sixty minutes before bed (blue light suppresses melatonin)
- Create a wind-down ritual to signal your nervous system that it's safe to rest
- Consider magnesium glycinate or a small protein-fat snack before bed if three a.m. wake-ups are your nemesis

(See **your Sleep & Sanity Support Kit** and **Wind Down Ritual Template** for step-by-step evening routines.)

Movement That Supports, Not Depletes

Exercise is a stressor, which can be good, but only if your body can recover from it. The goal here is to **build strength, not drain your reserves**.

- **Do:** strength training two to three times a week, daily walking, mobility work, and stretching
- **Do:** move in ways that feel good now, not just in ways that burn calories
- **Don't:** push through chronic cardio or high-intensity workouts if you're already feeling depleted (They'll only dig you deeper.)

When these four foundations are in place, your cells have:

- The raw materials (minerals) to function
- The steady fuel (blood sugar stability) to keep going

- The rest (sleep) to repair
- The movement signals to grow stronger

Everything else you add in the Middle and Top layers will take root more easily and *work the way they're supposed to.*

Middle Layer in Action: Targeted Support

Once your Base Layer is steady, it's time to start adding in targeted supports—the ones that address specific systems in your body that need extra attention right now.

Think of this layer like specialized tools in your toolbox. You don't need to use all of them at once, and some you may only need them for a season. These supports work best when guided by testing. If testing is not available and your symptoms clearly point to a system, start small and reassess. Pick only what matches your current priorities.

Liver Support

Your liver is the ultimate multitasker, filtering toxins, processing hormones, regulating blood sugar, and aiding digestion. But midlife can bring extra load: hormone shifts, environmental toxins, alcohol, medications, or past exposures (like mold) can all slow its capacity.

- Start your day with lemon water or add bitters before meals to boost bile flow.
- Eat cruciferous veggies (broccoli, cabbage, arugula, Brussels sprouts) several times a week.
- Use gentle detox tools like castor oil packs, sweating (sauna or exercise), or Epsom salt baths.
- Reduce exposure to toxins where you can. Switch to clean skincare and household products.

*(See your **Liver Support Toolkit** for step-by-step strategies and favorite recipes.)*

Hormone Balance

Your hormones are chemical messengers that impact everything from mood to metabolism. In midlife, small imbalances can create outsized symptoms, and supporting them can make a dramatic difference.

- Support progesterone (often low in midlife) with targeted drops or herbs, as guided by your practitioner
- Anchor your cortisol rhythm by getting morning light, reducing late-night screen time, and keeping blood sugar stable
- Support estrogen detox pathways with cruciferous veggies, adequate fiber, and liver support

If you've done DUTCH testing, use your results to pinpoint what needs the most support.

Digestion Optimization

If your digestion isn't working well, you won't absorb the nutrients you're working so hard to eat. Common signs you need digestive support: bloating, heartburn, constipation, loose stools, or feeling overly full after small meals.

- Use digestive enzymes with meals to help break down proteins, fats, and carbs
- Try digestive bitters or lemon water before meals to stimulate stomach acid
- Add probiotics (spore-based or strain-specific) as needed, based on symptoms or testing

*(Your **GI-MAP** test results can guide you to exactly which supports are right for you.)*

Nervous System Regulation

Your nervous system sets the tone for your entire body. If it's stuck in fight-or-flight, healing slows, hormones misfire, and digestion suffers.

- Practice daily breathwork (three to five minutes) to signal safety to your body
- Take unplugged breaks from screens and constant input
- Schedule "downshift" time (quiet walks, light stretching, or time in nature) especially at the end of your workday
- Consider a neuro panel for targeted support

*(See your **Sleep & Sanity Support Kit** for a full Nervous System Reset Toolkit.)*

Why This Layer Works Best After Foundations

If you jump straight into targeted supports without first shoring up your foundation, they won't work the way they're supposed to. A sluggish liver can't clear hormones efficiently if you're running on poor sleep and unstable blood sugar. Digestive enzymes can't do much if your cells don't have the minerals to fuel the process.

Targeted supports may be temporary—sometimes just a few months—and are best guided by testing so you're addressing your body's current priorities, not guessing.

Top Layer in Action: Lifestyle & Mindset Shifts

This is the layer where you turn progress into permanence. Your results stop being temporary fixes and start becoming your new normal. Without it, even the best foundations and targeted supports can slip away the moment life gets busy. These shifts aren't about doing *more,* they're about doing *what matters most,* consistently, so you stay aligned with your body instead of falling back into old patterns.

Prioritize Yourself Without Guilt

You are the engine of your life. If you run yourself into the ground, everything else slows down, too. Putting yourself on your own priority list isn't selfish; it's strategic. It means your health gets handled *before* the crisis point, so you can keep showing up for everyone and everything you care about.

Protect Your Energy Like a Business Asset

Time is finite, but energy is your most valuable currency. Boundaries protect it. Say "no" when you need to. Step back from commitments that drain you. Just like you wouldn't spend all your savings on a whim, don't spend all your energy on things that don't serve your health and joy.

Practice Body Trust Over Perfection

Midlife brings change. Some changes you can predict, some you can't. Trusting your body means you stop micromanaging every calorie or workout and start listening to what your body is telling you. This isn't about perfect adherence to a plan. It's about noticing patterns, responding early, and making choices that keep you feeling steady and strong.

Leverage the Ripple Effect

Small actions done consistently have a way of spilling over into every corner of your life. Drinking enough water can boost your energy, which improves your mood, which makes it easier to choose nourishing meals, which supports your sleep. And so it goes. Anchor a few keystone habits and let them create momentum for you.

Check In Before You Fall Back

Schedule regular lab rechecks (once a year, or sooner if new symptoms pop up) to catch changes early and protect the energy, clarity, and strength you've worked so hard for. In between, tune in to your body's early signals: sleep changes, mood shifts, unexplained weight fluctuations, or digestive changes. Address them before they snowball.

Here's the bottom line:

When you work the **Wellness Plan Pyramid** in order, each layer amplifies the one before it. Your foundations hold up your targeted supports. Your targeted supports work better when your mindset and lifestyle protect the progress you've made. Skip steps, and it's like swimming upstream. Build in order, and the current carries you forward.

Your Midlife Body Code Roadmap

Now that you've seen how the **Wellness Plan Pyramid works**, let's make it personal. I've created a one-page tool that walks you through building your own plan—step by step—so you know exactly where to start and what to focus on next.

Think of **Your Midlife Body Code Roadmap** as your quick-reference guide. It takes everything we've covered and distills it into a clear, simple action plan you can actually stick to—without the overwhelm.

Some women take this framework and run with it on their own. Others want an experienced guide in their corner—someone who can interpret test results, fine-tune the plan, and keep them accountable when life gets busy. Whichever path you choose, your Roadmap will keep you moving forward. And if you decide you want that guide, that's exactly the work I do with my clients every day.

🎁 Get Your Roadmap! Scan the QR code below or visit: https://YourMidlifeBodyCode.com/bonuses to download **Your Midlife Body Code Roadmap** and start mapping your next steps.

Whether you're moving forward solo or with support, there is one more piece to keep in mind before you dive in: the small but powerful habits can either keep you on track or quietly pull you off course. Your Roadmap gives you the structure. But structure alone isn't enough. You also need to know what can quietly derail your progress so you can steer clear.

Common Pitfalls That Stall Progress

Even with the best plan, a few sneaky habits can quietly derail your momentum. Keep an eye out for these:

- **Letting boundaries slide:** saying yes when you need to say no, and draining your energy reserves in the process
- **Underfueling:** skipping protein or going too long without eating, leaving your blood sugar on a rollercoaster
- **Ignoring small signals:** brushing off new symptoms instead of addressing them early

- **Falling into "all-or-nothing" mode:** pushing too hard, burning out, and stopping completely instead of adjusting and continuing

Your best defense? Stay rooted in your foundations. When you keep those steady, these pitfalls don't stand a chance.

Client Case Study: Beverly's Pyramid in Action

When Beverly came to me, she was stuck in a frustrating pattern. For years, she'd been dealing with what doctors called "chronic UTIs," cycling on and off antibiotics every few months, only to have the symptoms return. Her energy crashed mid-afternoon, her sleep was never truly restorative, and despite her clean diet and intense workouts, she couldn't shake the stubborn weight.

Beverly was a high-achieving, type A professional who didn't know how to slow down. Her job was high-pressure, and she "managed" it by pushing herself harder at work, in the gym, and in life. Her HTMA told the story her body had been trying to communicate for years: a calcium shell, signaling her nervous system had been locked in overdrive for far too long. Add in mold-related toxicity, gut imbalances, and nervous system dysregulation, and her system was tapped out.

In the past, she might have jumped straight into gut protocols or mold detox. This time, we honored the **Wellness Plan Pyramid**.

Step 1—Base Layer

We started by giving her body the raw materials and safety signals it needed:

- Adrenal support and mineral-rich foods to rebuild potassium and magnesium and reabsorb lost calcium

- Higher-protein meals earlier in the day to stabilize blood sugar
- A wind-down routine that helped her body downshift at night
- Swapping overly intense, high-demand workouts for strength training, walking, and stretching so her nervous system could finally take a breather

Within weeks, her energy was more stable, her sleep deepened, and she felt less on edge.

Step 2—Middle Layer

Once her foundation was solid, we layered in targeted supports:

- Gut repair nutrients to improve digestion and reduce inflammation
- Nervous system regulation practices to keep her out of constant "go mode"
- A gentle, phased mold detox protocol, which, after completing, finally ended her years-long cycle of chronic UTI symptoms.

Once her body wasn't stuck in crisis mode, the things we added worked, and the changes started to last.

Step 3—Top Layer

Finally, Beverly built in the lifestyle and mindset shifts that would support and keep her progress:

- Saying no to overcommitting her time and energy
- Protecting space for rest and recovery
- Listening to her body's cues instead of overriding them with willpower

Beverly went from feeling like her health was a full-time job to feeling steady, capable, and in control of her body again.

Takeaway: Why This Worked

Beverly didn't "fix" herself with one supplement or quick protocol. She worked in the right order:

- **Base first** so her body had the fuel and safety to shift out of survival mode
- **Middle next** so targeted supports could actually work
- **Top last** so lifestyle and mindset changes could lock it all in

When you build in order, your body doesn't have to fight you. It works with you.

Reader Reflection

Take a moment to look at your own **Wellness Plan Pyramid**.

- Which layer are you focused on right now, Base, Middle, or Top?
- Are you tempted to skip ahead like Beverly once did, or are you giving your body the support it needs in the order it needs it?
- If you could make just *one* change this week that your future self would thank you for, what would it be?

Write it in your journal or on your **Midlife Body Code Roadmap**. Small, well-placed steps compound into big change faster than you think.

Your Next Layer

You don't have to do everything at once to make progress. In fact, the women who see the biggest wins are the ones who start small, stay consistent, and build in order. Even if you're not doing functional testing right now, you can still make powerful changes. Support your nervous system, stabilize your blood sugar, and give your liver the raw materials it needs. You might be surprised how much shifts just from that foundation.

Remember, this isn't about perfection. It's about alignment—doing what serves your body best at this moment. The **Midlife Body Code** isn't just a program; it's a lifelong framework you can return to and refine as your body changes. You've decoded and realigned. Now it's about continuing to reclaim, layer by layer.

You've built your **Wellness Plan Pyramid** from the ground up, layering in the right supports at the right time. You've learned how to read your body's signals, respond with what it truly needs, and adjust as you go. This isn't about chasing youth, it's about stepping into midlife with clarity, strength, and energy you can count on.

Next, we move beyond fixing what is wrong and into what it means to thrive: a life not just free of symptoms, but rich with energy, purpose, and joy.

TL;DR—Chapter 12: Building Your Functional Wellness Plan

- Real progress comes from structure, not overwhelm. Work the Wellness Plan Pyramid from the ground up.
- Base Layer: Minerals, blood sugar balance, quality sleep, and movement that strengthens without draining.
- Middle Layer: Targeted supports (hormones, liver, digestion, nervous system) added strategically after the foundation is steady.

- Top Layer: Lifestyle and mindset shifts—boundaries, body trust, and regular check-ins—that make progress sustainable.
- Each layer amplifies the one below it; skip steps and progress slips, build in order and momentum carries you forward.

Bottom line: Lasting results don't come from doing everything. They come from doing the right things in the right order.

Conclusion: Thriving in Midlife. You Hold the Key

Midlife isn't the end of the story; it's the turning point. It's the season when you finally get to write the script on your terms, not based on old rules that never worked for you in the first place.

Thriving in midlife doesn't mean chasing who you were at twenty-five. It means finally feeling at home in your body again and having the energy, clarity, and calm to enjoy it.

You've already decoded the old patterns that kept you stuck. Now, you get to let them go. Let's set the record straight about what thriving really means. For too long, women have been fed outdated, punishing definitions of health and success.

- Health ≠ extreme dieting
- Success ≠ pushing through exhaustion
- Worth ≠ shrinking your body

That narrative ends here.

This next chapter of your life isn't about fitting into someone else's mold. **It's about feeling good in your skin, living with energy that lasts, and reclaiming the confidence that comes when you're aligned with your body instead of fighting it.**

The New Definition of Normal

For too long, women have been told that feeling worse with every passing year is just part of "getting older." But that isn't normal. And it certainly isn't your destiny.

Normal is *not*:

- Constant bloating, fatigue, irritability, and brain fog
- Accepting that this is just "getting older"
- Feeling disconnected from your body

Your new normal is:

- Being proactive, not reactive
- Feeling empowered, not overwhelmed
- Knowing your body's needs and responding with care

You get to decide what normal feels like for you—not your doctor, not the wellness industry, not even your past self. You've begun to realign your daily choices with what your body truly needs. And that alignment creates a steady, sustainable rhythm that supports your energy, mood, and clarity day after day.

Maintaining Your Midlife Body Code (Without Obsessing)

You do not need to be perfect to feel good. What matters is consistency, not control. The goal is progress and alignment, not chasing some unrealistic ideal. When you show up for yourself in small but steady ways, your body responds with more energy, balance, and clarity.

Here are simple strategies that make this sustainable:

- Regular check-ins with your energy, mood, and digestion
- Staying consistent with foundational habits like adding in minerals, balanced blood sugar, and quality sleep
- Adjusting with life's seasons, whether that means travel, busy schedules, or shifting hormones

This is not a thirty-day challenge; it becomes your way of living. It is how you reclaim lasting energy and confidence without obsession.

The Real Win: Trusting Yourself Again

Energy, weight, and mood matter. But the real win is trusting yourself again. When you started this journey, you may have felt like your body was fighting you at every turn. Now you know how to listen to its signals, respond with care, and feel confident in the choices you make. That self-trust is what changes everything.

Here's what it can look like in real life:

- **Yolanda:** "I feel happy every morning. I wake up with energy. I'm getting my strength back in my whole body." She's no longer letting overwhelm control her days. Instead, she has the energy and resilience to be present with her granddaughters.
- **Janice:** "This is the FIRST week I've had multiple days in a row when I have had my brain back! As of Monday, I can track things again!" She once thought her only option was pushing harder at the gym. Now, she listens to her body's cues and gets results without burnout.
- **Colleen:** "It's a long road, but I know I'm building a solid foundation. It's not a quick fix, but I'm starting to feel like things are aligning. My joints aren't hurting after activities that usually lead to pain. I'm staying asleep more often and feeling less brain fog." And what's more, she finally trusts the process—and her body—again.
- **Dana:** She used to plan her day around bathroom stops. Now she can go out to eat, laugh with friends, and enjoy a meal without worrying if she'll need to run to the restroom. That freedom gave her back confidence she didn't realize she'd lost.

- **Hannah:** "I have more energy, my aches and pains are gone, and my sleep is improved." She even lost eighteen pounds in six months without dieting, but for her, the real win was finally feeling well enough to enjoy life again.
- **Jessica:** "My knees don't hurt! We walked flights of stairs, and somehow, they still don't hurt." Sometimes the biggest wins show up in the simple things you can now do with ease.
- **Lenora:** "My hair feels so much better!! What is going on? All of a sudden, it feels fuller and lush!" Beyond the cosmetic change, her story shows how deep repair creates vitality in unexpected places.

These everyday wins are proof that it is not about perfection; it is about reclaiming your confidence in your body. You've gone from frustration to clarity, from doubt to certainty. And that shift changes everything.

You are the CEO of Your Health

When you began this journey, you may have felt like a passenger in your own body. You were waiting for answers, waiting for energy to come back, waiting for someone else to tell you what was wrong. That waiting is over.

Now you know how to read your body's signals, interpret data, and make decisions that support real progress. You've stepped into the CEO role. A CEO doesn't do everything herself. She sets the vision, weighs the information in front of her, and makes informed choices. You are now doing the same for your health.

This doesn't mean going it alone. It means being informed, empowered, and supported by the right partners so you can continue to move forward with clarity. The real freedom comes when you know you are not at the mercy of symptoms or rushed appointments anymore. You're back in the driver's seat and you're not giving up that seat again. You are the CEO of your health story, fully capable of leading your body into its next chapter.

Continuing Your Midlife Body Code Journey

If you're ready to go deeper, more support and tools are waiting for you. Whether that means exploring functional testing, building more tailored protocols, or having a trusted guide to walk beside you, support is available when you are ready to step back into your power.

Remember, reclaiming your health isn't about perfection; it's about progress. Every step you take builds on the last, and you now have the tools to keep moving forward. You've just learned the **Midlife Body Code** Method. If you want to keep decoding, realigning, and reclaiming, visit https://YourMidlifeBody Code.com/bonuses_to join the community and access the resources that will help you keep moving forward.

You Hold the Key

This isn't the end of your journey; it's the beginning of something bigger. Midlife isn't a time to shrink back. It's your time to rise, thrive, and show up with the impact, energy, and joy that have always been yours to claim.

What thriving in midlife really feels like:

- Steady, sustainable energy without the crash and burn
- Clear-headed focus and emotional steadiness
- Deep, restorative sleep and smooth digestion
- The ability to move through life with ease and presence
- Confidence in listening to and trusting your body's signals

- Living in alignment with your body rather than fighting against it

You've already seen what this looks like for women like Jessica, Colleen, and Lenora. Their transformations remind you that these shifts are possible, no matter how stuck you may feel today. Now it's your turn. You've decoded your body's signals, and you know how to respond. Midlife is no longer something to *endure*. It's a *season to claim* with **energy, clarity, and confidence**.

The code isn't hidden—you've had the key all along. Now you know how to use it. This isn't just the framework for this book; it's your lifelong compass.

Decode. Realign. Reclaim.

Because midlife isn't the end of your story. It's the beginning of your power.

TL;DR—Conclusion: Thriving in Midlife. You Hold the Key

- Thriving in midlife means feeling at home in your body— not chasing your twenty-five-year-old self.
- Your new normal is proactive, empowered, and aligned with your body—not suffering with brain fog, fatigue, or bloat.
- Progress, not perfection, keeps you steady. Foundations like minerals, blood sugar, and sleep create momentum.
- The real win is trusting yourself again.
- You are the CEO of your health, leading with clarity, confidence, and choice.
- The code isn't hidden. You've had the key all along.

This is not the end of your journey. It's your lifelong compass: Decode. Realign. Reclaim.

Final Word

You've faced the frustration, pushed past the noise, and found your way back to your own voice. That's not luck. That's power. You now have the tools, the knowledge, and the trust in yourself to lead your body forward in a way that works for *you*.

There's no more waiting for the "right time" or the "perfect plan." **You are the plan.**

You decide what thriving looks like.

You know how to create it—and you're not asking for permission.

Your best chapter starts now. And you're the one writing every word—bold, clear, and entirely your own. This isn't about going back to who you were. It's about becoming the most vibrant, capable, unapologetic version of yourself yet. **Midlife is not your fade-out. It's your rise.**

Resources

Your journey doesn't end with this book. If you're ready to go deeper, these resources—books, websites, and experts—can help you expand your knowledge, find new perspectives, and keep building momentum on your midlife health journey. I've grouped them by topic so you can quickly find what feels most relevant to you right now.

Your Tools & Next Steps

Bonus Resources Portal—All the practical trackers, guides, and templates mentioned throughout the book, all in one place.
☞ https://YourMidlifeBodyCode.com/bonuses

Bye-Bye Stubborn Weight Meal Plan—A free plan to help you balance blood sugar and fuel your body for sustainable energy and weight release.
☞ https://YourMidlifeBodyCode.com/bye-bye

Root Cause Lab Review—A one-on-one review of your existing blood labs through a functional lens (with a special reader discount code).

☞ https://YourMidlifeBodyCode.com/lab-review

Menopause & Hormones

Haver, Mary Claire. *The New Menopause: Navigating Your Path Through Hormonal Change with Purpose, Power, and Facts.* Rodale Books, 2024.

Fadal, Tamsen. *How to Menopause: Take Charge of Your Health, Reclaim Your Life, and Feel Even Better Than Before.* Grand Central Publishing, 2025.

Vitti, Alisa. *In the Flo: Unlock Your Hormonal Advantage and Revolutionize Your Life.* HarperOne, 2020.

The Menopause Society. *Menopause Society.*
https://menopause.org/ The Menopause Society
(This is the site formerly known as the North American Menopause Society.)

Blood Sugar & Metabolism

Means, Casey (with Calley Means). *Good Energy: The Surprising Connection Between Metabolism and Limitless Health.* Avery / Penguin Random House, 2024.

Inchauspé, Jessie. **Glucose Revolution**: *The Life-Changing Power of Balancing Your Blood Sugar*. Simon Element, 2022.

Mold & Environmental Health

Nathan, Neil, and Robert K. Naviaux. **Toxic**: *Heal Your Body from Mold Toxicity, Lyme Disease, Multiple Chemical Sensitivities, and Chronic Environmental Illness*. Victory Belt Publishing, 2018 (2nd Edition in 2025).

Crista, Jill. **Break the Mold**: *5 Tools to Conquer Mold and Take Back Your Health*. Wellness Ink Publishing, 2018.

Carnahan, Jill, M.D. "Resources Roadmap." *Dr. Jill Carnahan,* https://www.jillcarnahan.com/resources-roadmap/

Additional Mold Resources:
- Environmental Protection Agency: https://www.epa.gov/mold
- Centers for Disease Control: https://www.cdc.gov/mold/default.htm
- IICRC website (for remediation resources): https://iicrc.org/

Brain Health & Cognition

Naidoo, Uma. **This Is Your Brain on Food**: *An Indispensable Guide to the Surprising Foods That Fight Depression, Anxiety, PTSD, OCD, ADHD, and More*. Little, Brown Spark, 2020.

Naidoo, Uma. **Calm Your Mind with Food**: *A Revolutionary Guide to Controlling Your Anxiety*. Bloomsbury Publishing, 2023

Chapman, Angela, M.Ed., FDN. *Anti-Alzheimer's: What Your Doctor Hasn't Told You About the Prevention and Reversal of Cognitive Decline.* CreateSpace Independent Publishing Platform, 2017.

Breathwork & Nervous System Regulation

Nestor, James. *Breath: The New Science of a Lost Art.* Riverhead Books, 2020.

Singer, Michael A. *The Untethered Soul: The Journey Beyond Yourself.* New Harbinger Publications, 2007.

Habib, Navaz, M.D. *Activate Your Vagus Nerve: Unleash Your Body's Natural Ability to Heal.* Ulysses Press, 2019.

Gut Health & Nutrition

Bulsiewicz, Will. *Fiber Fueled: The Plant-Based Gut Health Program for Losing Weight, Restoring Your Health, and Optimizing Your Microbiome.* Avery, 2020.

Olien, Darin. *SuperLife: The 5 Simple Fixes That Will Make You Healthy, Fit, and Eternally Awesome.* Rodale Books, 2017.

Rossi, Megan. *Love Your Gut: Supercharge Your Digestive Health and Transform Your Wellbeing.* Penguin Life, 2020.

Women's Empowerment

Rodsky, Eve. *Find Your Unicorn Space: Reclaim Your Creative Life in a Too-Busy World.* G.P. Putnam's Sons, 2022.

Nagoski, Emily, and Amelia Nagoski. *Burnout: The Secret to Unlocking the Stress Cycle.* Ballantine Books, 2019.

Edden, Jenn. **Woman Unleashed**: *The Highly Sensitive Woman's Guide to Radiant Energy, Unstoppable Confidence, and a 21-Day Plan to Kick Sugar's Hold on You.* You Speak It Publishing, 2016.

Remember, information is powerful, but only when you use it. Choose one next step, one resource, or one practice to lean into today, and let it remind you that your midlife body is not broken, it's ready to be decoded, realigned, and reclaimed.

Sending you so much love!
Claudine
Your Midlife Body Code Expert

Acknowledgements

This is my first book (who knows what the future holds!), and I was woefully unprepared for what it takes to turn an idea into something tangible you can hold in your hands. I could not have done it without so many people, but the first person to really see this project and believe in it wholeheartedly was my publisher, Cori Wamsley. She answered my many (many, many!) questions, gave me practical feedback, and kept me accountable. Thank you, Cori, for guiding me and for helping me get this book into the hands of the women who need it most.

I also had the privilege of some amazing pre-readers—Jennifer Shepherd, Krista Beavers, Melanie White, LeTasha Souffrant, and Cristina Francois—who gave their time, thoughtful feedback, and encouragement. Your insights shaped this book more than you know, and I am deeply grateful.

To my parents, my sisters, my children, and my husband: every lesson, every conversation, and every ounce of love helped shape this woman who now believes we can repair our bodies when we give them the right tools. Thank you for standing by me in ways both big and small.

To my dear friends Jenn Edden and Brandie Tselekidis: thank you for being my sounding boards, for propping me up, and for always making me laugh.

To the incredible women I've had the privilege to work with: thank you for trusting me with your stories. Your courage to share, to do the work, and to reclaim your health has inspired every page of this book.

To the FDN course and community: thank you for giving me the knowledge and support to step into this work. A special thank you to Sarah Ball for introducing me to this world, and to my mentors Brandon Mollé and Lisa Pitel-Killah, who have taught me more than I ever imagined I could learn.

To my many coaches and mentors over the years—especially Danielle DeAnna, Allyson Chavez, Joie Gharrity, and Alison

Haugan—thank you for believing in me, for challenging me, and for quietly pushing me to grow even when I resisted.

For the heavy lifting on the production side, I must thank my editor, Allison Hrip, and cover designer, Karen Captline. Working with a first-time author is no easy task, and your patience, creativity, and care helped bring this vision to life. You are absolute gems.

And finally, to my husband Brent, who deserves more than just a line or two here. While I poured nights and weekends into this labor of love, he made dinners, did dishes, drove the kids, and carried the weight of everything else so I could carry this. Brent, you are my partner in every sense of the word. I could not have done this without your love, support, and unwavering belief in me.

About Claudine

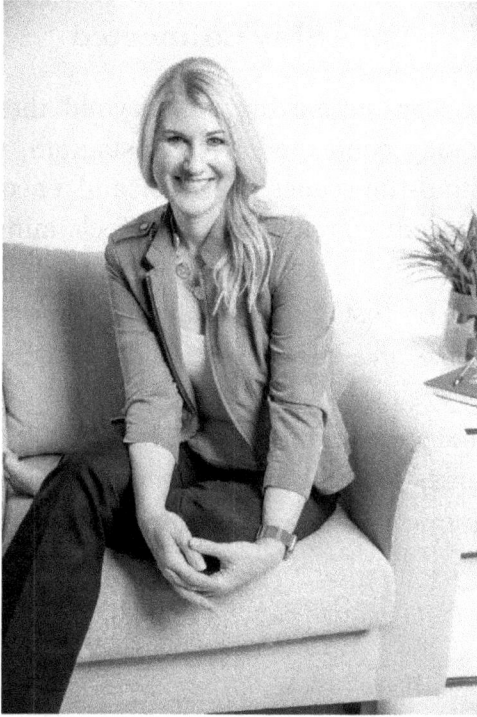

Claudine François is a board-certified functional medicine and holistic health practitioner and the creator of The Midlife Body Code Method. A former CFO turned root-cause detective, she helps driven women over forty uncover the hidden reasons behind exhaustion, stubborn weight, brain fog, digestive struggles, thyroid imbalances, and hormone shifts.

Through advanced functional labs and personalized protocols, Claudine guides women to decode their symptoms, realign with their bodies, and reclaim lasting energy, clarity, and vitality—without extreme diets, dismissive doctors, or endless trial-and-error.

Her book, *Your Midlife Body Code*, expands on her proven method to empower women to finally feel heard, understand their bodies, and take back control of their health in midlife and beyond.

Let's Stay Connected

I'd love to keep supporting you beyond these pages. The easiest way to stay connected is on Instagram, where I share fresh tips, behind-the-scenes insights, and encouragement to help you keep decoding, realigning, and reclaiming *your* Midlife Body Code.

☞ Follow me on Instagram: @claudine.r.francois

If you'd like deeper dives and functional medicine walkthroughs, you can also find me on YouTube: www.youtube.com/@claudinefrancois1026.

And of course, you'll always find my latest tools, programs, and updates on my website: www.ingoodcleantaste.com.

Index

Body Systems & Functions

Additional Terms